DR. LUNA O. RICHARDS

CHRONIC
KIDNEY DISEASE
STAGE 3
Cookbook
for WOMEN

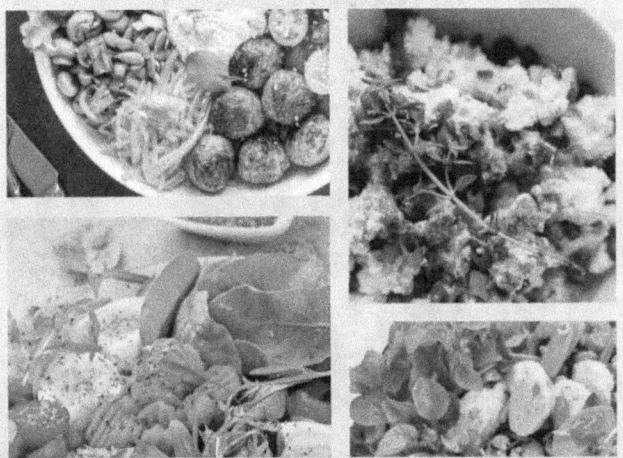

Quick and Easy Low Sodium, Low Potassium, and Low
Phosphorus Recipes & Meal Plan For Stage 3 Kidney Disease
Diet (CKD) for Managing Kidney Disease and Avoiding Dialysis

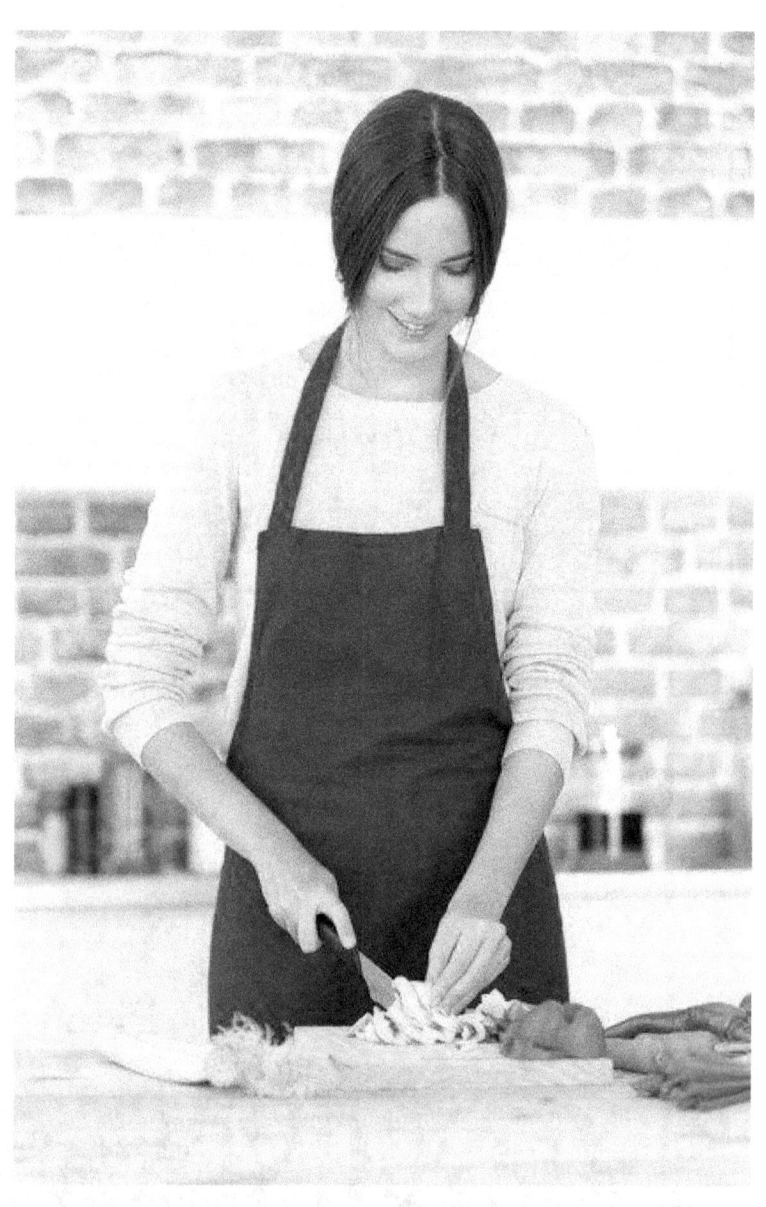

Dedication

This book *"Chronic Kidney Disease Stage 3 Cookbook for Women"* is dedicated to each and every woman out there fighting for survival. May this book bring forth a renewed hope in yourhealing journey.

This book is a work of *"personalized experience"* and it willsurely be a guide to your wellness.

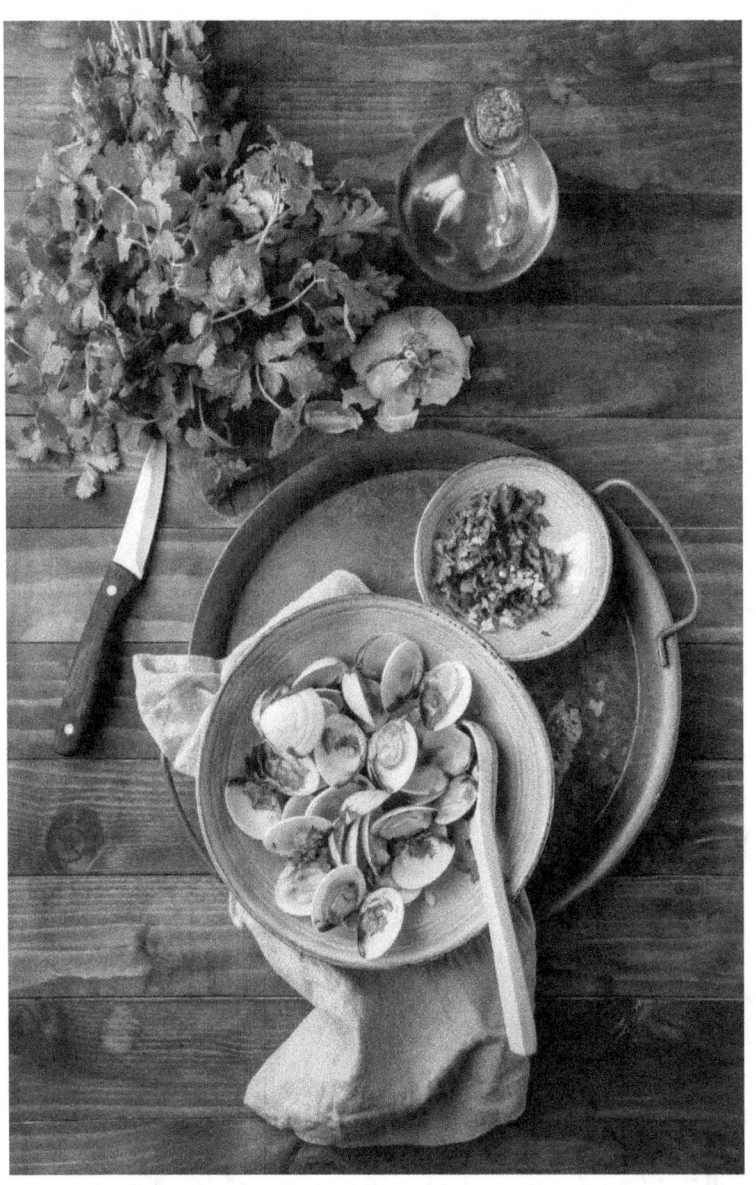

Table of Contents

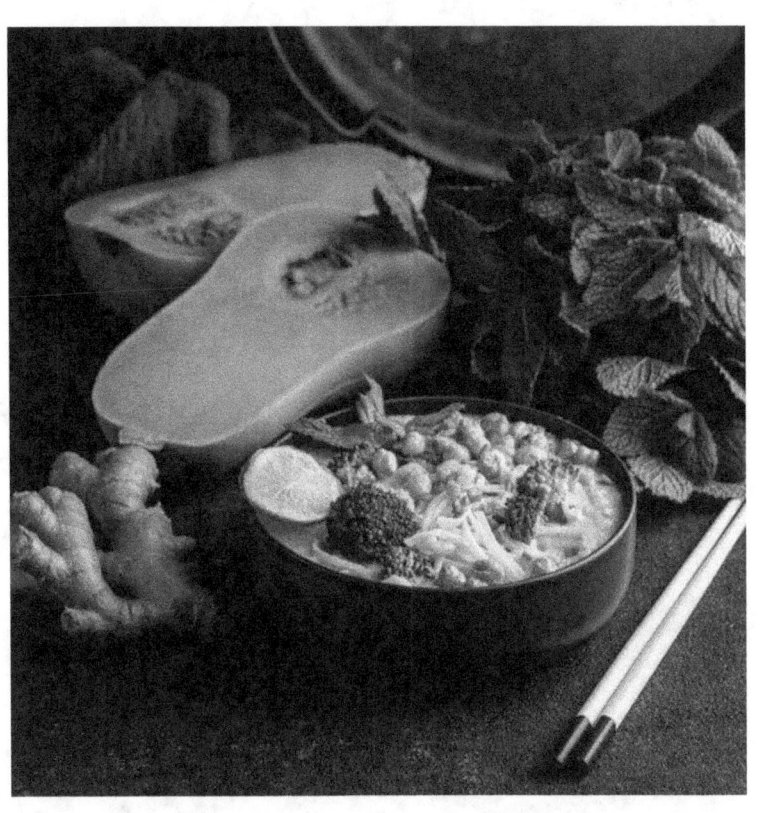

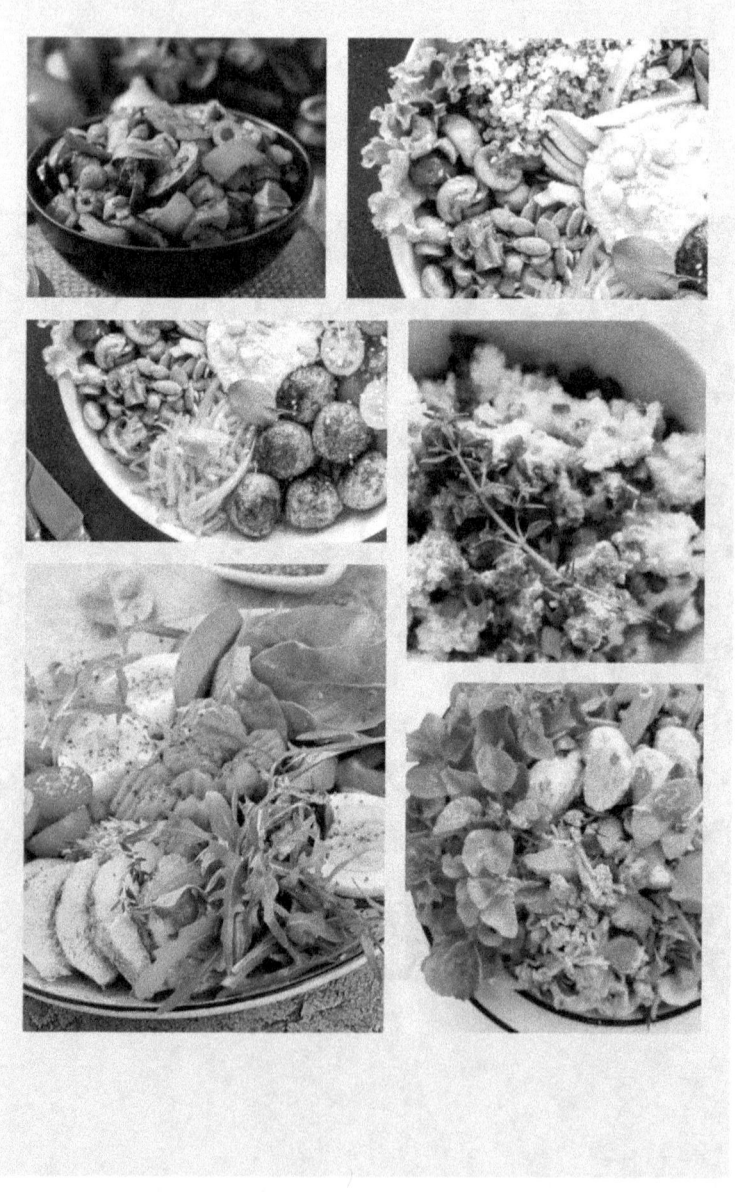

A Survivor's Story

My name is Rose, I used to have a friend named Betty. Today I will be sharing the transformative journey of Betty's Chronic Kidney Disease Stage 3.

Betty was once caught up in the whirlwind of life's demands, striving to juggle her career as an accountant while nurturing a family. Her days were consumed by the relentless pace of work, leaving little room for the simple joys of home. Despite her dedication, the echoes of her late returns, a byproduct of her commitment to her profession, echoed in the silence of her familial bonds.

The strains of a demanding job and a deteriorating relationship gradually gnawed at the fabric of her marriage. Arguments ignited like sparks in the night, fueled by the flickering absence that Betty's late hours cast upon her home.

Regrettably, her marriage, once the cornerstone of her happiness, crumbled under the weight of missed connections and unmet expectations.

With the gavel of divorce echoing in the chambers of her life, Betty found herself in a realm of uncharted territory. She found herself staring helplessly in the corridors of depression, with no one to fall back on, Betty confided in alcohol and cigarettes, to ease away her agony. A single mother facing the trials of raising her children alone, her days became an unyielding battle to meet their needs, leaving scant time for self-care or nourishing meals. As the stressors mounted, her emotional state began to crumble, and her diet suffered, becoming a casualty of her overwhelming responsibilities.

Months passed in a haze of relentless obligations, and whispers of illness began to manifest in Betty's body. Lingering fatigue, persistent discomfort, and a deep-seated weariness crept into her daily existence. A visit to the hospital unraveled the unwelcome truth: Chronic Kidney

Disease had woven its invisible threads into the fabric of her being.

Betty stood at the precipice of uncertainty, grappling with the weight of this diagnosis. Yet, amid the shadows, a glimmer of hope emerged. In a chance conversation at work, she confided in a colleague who, with empathy and understanding, guided her towards a beacon of light—a dedicated dietitian.

In the comforting space of the dietician's office, Betty found solace and direction. The dietitian, understanding the importance of nutrition in managing CKD, introduced Betty to the *"Chronic Kidney Disease Cookbook Stage 3."* With trembling hands and a heart heavy with apprehension, she ventured into the world of nourishing recipes and kidney-friendly meals.

Armed with the guidance from the cookbook, Betty embarked on a transformative journey. With each page turned, she discovered a newfound passion for preparing wholesome, kidney-supportive meals. These kidney-friendly diet supported her kidney health by reducing workload, managing blood pressure, regulating electrolytes, moderating protein intake, and balancing fluid levels. Slowly but steadily, her kitchen became an oasis of healing, filled with the aromas of nourishment and the promise of better health.

In the embrace of this cookbook's guidance, Betty witnessed subtle yet significant changes. Her body responded to the kindness of nutritious meals, and a sense of vitality rekindled within her. The burden of managing her condition felt lighter as she embraced the nourishing power of food tailored for her kidneys.

Betty's story is one of resilience, courage, and the transformative influence of nutrition on her journey through chronic kidney disease. With the aid of the cookbook and the compassionate guidance of her dietitian, Betty found not just sustenance but a pathway towards reclaiming her health and well-being.

Introduction

Welcome to *"Chronic Kidney Disease Stage 3 for Women".* Are you ready to embrace a life where nourishment becomes your ally in managing Chronic Kidney Disease Stage 3? This cookbook isn't just a collection of recipes; it's a compassionate guide crafted to empower women in their fight against this condition while savoring every flavorful bite."

As a seasoned dietitian and advocate for holistic health, I've witnessed firsthand the significance of a tailored diet in managing chronic kidney disease. My passion stems from guiding countless individuals, especially women, through this challenging phase, witnessing their resilience and triumphs.

Imagine feeling empowered, not overwhelmed, by the choices on your plate. Imagine relishing meals that are both delicious and specifically designed to support your kidney health. I've seen the transformative impact of nutrition on managing CKD Stage 3, fostering hope and strength among my patients.

This cookbook is not merely a culinary collection; it's a vital tool in navigating the intricate landscape of Chronic Kidney Disease Stage 3. Each recipe has been meticulously crafted, balancing taste with nutritional integrity, catering specifically to the unique dietary needs of women managing this condition.

From my professional standpoint, I firmly believe that food is medicine. With the right guidance, nourishing meals can play a pivotal role in enhancing vitality and mitigating the progression of CKD Stage 3. This book stands as a testament to this belief, offering a multitude of recipes tailored to optimize kidney health.

This comprehensive guide dives deep into the nuances of managing CKD Stage 3 for women. From insightful explanations about the disease's biochemistry to an array of mouthwatering recipes specifically curated to be kidney-friendly, this book leaves no stone unturned. It offers meal plans, grocery lists, and practical tips for effective dietary management, ensuring ease and convenience.

Delve into this book and discover the art of crafting delicious meals while safeguarding your kidney health. Uncover the secrets behind meal planning, grocery shopping tips, and learn how to create tantalizing dishes without sacrificing taste or health. Banish the fear of bland diets; these recipes are a celebration of flavors tailored to suit your needs, promising an exciting culinary journey.

Are you ready to embark on a gastronomic adventure that nourishes your body, tantalizes your taste buds, and empowers your journey towards wellness? This cookbook is not just about recipes; it's a beacon of hope, offering guidance, support, and above all, delicious meals that elevate your health.

Join me as we savor the flavors of life, one kidney-friendly recipe at a time.

Remember, health starts from within – and it begins on your plate. Let's cook our way to vibrant health together!

Flip through the pages as you enjoy your read!

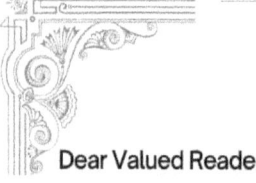

Dear Valued Reader,

Thank you for selecting our cookbook from among the many available. Your decision to live a healthy lifestyle with the help of our book means everything to us. We welcome you to share your thoughts on the website by leaving a polite review. Your feedback supports our journey, and we are grateful. Let your words be the heartbeat of our collective dedication to happiness. We also humbly request that you visit and follow our author page; by doing so, you will be exposed to a plethora of other publications by this author.

With appreciation,

DR. LUNA O. RICHARDS

Part One

Understanding Chronic Kidney Disease Stage 3 in Women.

Chronic Kidney Disease (CKD) is a progressive condition characterized by the gradual loss of kidney function over time. When compared to previous stages, the kidneys in Stage 3 CKD show considerable impairment and a decline in their ability to filter waste and excess fluids from the circulation. Here's a biochemical rundown of what transpires in our system as women when diagnosed with CKD Stage 3:

The Biochemistry of CKD Stage 3 in Women

Understanding what happens in our bodies as women is the first step to healing and recovery in the midst of uncertainty; Changes in biochemical markers and physical processes occur as a result of diminishing kidney function in chronic kidney disease (CKD) Stage 3. Below we will evaluate several changes which occurs within us as a result of CKD Stage 3 disease:

1. **Reduced Glomerular Filtration Rate (GFR):** In Stage 3 CKD, GFR, a measure of renal function, decreases. Waste products (urea, creatinine) build in the blood as kidney function declines because they are not adequately filtered out.

2. **Electrolyte Imbalance:** Kidneys aid in the regulation of electrolytes such as potassium, sodium, and calcium. Electrolyte balance can be altered in CKD Stage 3, resulting in high potassium (hyperkalemia), low calcium, and high phosphate levels. This has the potential to affect bone health, muscular function, and heart rhythm.

3. **Acid-Base Balance:** The kidneys help to maintain the body's acid-base balance. Acid levels may rise when kidney

function declines, resulting to metabolic acidosis. This can result in exhaustion, confusion, and other symptoms.

4. **Anemia:** In CKD, a decrease in the synthesis of erythropoietin (a hormone produced by the kidneys) can result in anemia. Reduced red blood cell production has an impact on oxygen transport to tissues, contributing to weariness and weakness.

5. **Changes in Hormones:** The kidneys also regulate hormones such as vitamin D, which is necessary for bone health. Vitamin D levels may be insufficient in Stage 3 CKD, resulting in bone issues.

6. **Increased Blood Pressure:** CKD can contribute to elevated blood pressure, which further damages and aggravates the condition, producing a vicious cycle of decreasing renal function.

7. **Proteinuria:** Proteinuria (the presence of protein in the urine) is a sign of renal impairment in CKD. This may worsen as CKD progresses, increasing the risk of cardiovascular problems and hastening the deterioration of renal function.

CKD is categorized into five phases based on the estimated Glomerular Filtration Rate (eGFR), a measure of how well the kidneys filter waste from the blood. Stage 3 is subdivided into two substages: 3a and 3b, which are defined by the range of eGFR levels.

CKD Stage 3 is distinguished by significant renal impairment and an eGFR of 30-59 mL/min/1.73m2. Stages 3a (eGFR 45-59 mL/min/1.73m2) and 3b (eGFR 30-44 mL/min/1.73m2) show varying degrees of renal function deterioration.

The progression of Stage 3 CKD is frequently gradual and insidious. Patients may not exhibit apparent symptoms at first. However, as kidney function deteriorates more, symptoms such as weariness, swelling (edema), changes in urine frequency, and high blood pressure may appear.

Although both men and women are affected by CKD, certain variables may predispose women to a higher risk of kidney disease. According to certain research, autoimmune illnesses, urinary tract infections, pregnancy-related problems such as preeclampsia, and hormonal variations may all raise the risk of CKD in women.

Development of CKD Stage 3 in Women

1. **Underlying Causes:** Diabetes, high blood pressure (hypertension), glomerulonephritis, polycystic kidney disease, urinary tract blockages, and systemic disorders such as lupus are all risk factors for CKD. These disorders gradually weaken the kidneys, causing CKD to proceed.

2. **Progression:** As CKD progresses to Stage 3, kidney function deteriorates, reducing the organ's ability to filter

waste and excess fluids. This can lead to waste product accumulation in the blood, electrolyte abnormalities, and issues affecting other organ systems.

3. **Complications:** Complications associated with CKD Stage 3 include anemia, bone disease, cardiovascular issues, and fluid retention. Women with CKD may experience reproductive health complications such as menstruation abnormalities or infertility.

4. **Management and Treatment:** Treatment goals include slowing the progression of renal disease, managing symptoms, and preventing consequences. As kidney function falls, this includes lifestyle changes (dietary changes, exercise), regulating underlying illnesses, drugs, and, in certain cases, sophisticated procedures such as dialysis or kidney transplantation.

5. **Monitoring and Follow-up:** It is critical to assess the progression of CKD and alter treatment strategies based on

regular monitoring of renal function by blood tests, urine tests, and check-ups.

Causes of Stage 3 CKD in Women

Chronic Kidney Disease (CKD) Stage 3 in women can be caused by a variety of circumstances, including both causes similar to those seen in males and some unique to women. Understanding these reasons aids in the better identification and management of CKD in female patients:

1. **Diabetes:** This is the major cause of CKD in both men and women. Uncontrolled high blood sugar levels can damage the blood vessels in the kidneys and decrease their function over time.

2. **Hypertension (High Blood Pressure):** Another major cause of CKD is persistently high blood pressure. It puts strain on the blood arteries in the kidneys, causing injury and a gradual loss in function.

3. **Glomerulonephritis:** This disorder is characterized by inflammation of the filtration units (glomeruli) of the kidney. It can be caused by infections, autoimmune illnesses, or other systemic problems, and it can lead to kidney damage and CKD.

4. **Polycystic Kidney Disease (PKD):** PKD is a hereditary condition that causes many cysts to form in the kidneys, resulting in enlargement and ultimately function impairment. Women who have PKD may be at an increased risk of developing CKD.

5. **Urinary Tract Obstructions:** Conditions such as kidney stones, tumors, or congenital anomalies can obstruct the urinary tract, eventually resulting in reduced kidney function and CKD.

6. **Autoimmune disorders:** Autoimmune disorders such as lupus (systemic lupus erythematosus) or vasculitis can affect

the kidneys, causing inflammation and damage that eventually leads to CKD.

7. **Reproductive Factors:** Certain reproductive health issues, such as frequent urinary tract infections, kidney complications during pregnancy (such as preeclampsia), and complications due to certain drugs during pregnancy, may raise the risk of CKD in women.

8. **Other Factors:** Smoking, obesity, a family history of renal disease, and certain medications (for example, nonsteroidal anti-inflammatory drugs - NSAIDs) can all contribute to the development and progression of CKD in women.

Types of CKD Stage 3 That Women Should Know

CKD is classified into distinct categories based on the underlying reasons, which impact the kidneys differently. Here's an in-depth look at the many forms of CKD:

1. **Diabetes-Related Nephropathy:** This occurs as a result of diabetes mellitus complications, primarily type 1 or type 2 diabetes. In this condition, high blood sugar levels damage the blood arteries in the kidneys, causing kidney damage and impairment. Patients are likely to observe proteinuria (protein in the urine) and hypertension. It is the most common cause of end-stage kidney disease (ESKD).

2. **Nephropathy Due to Hypertension:** This arises as a result of uncontrolled high blood pressure over an extended period of time which goes further to destroy the blood vessels in the kidneys. Chronic hypertension strains the arteries, resulting in decreased blood flow and, eventually,

kidney injury. Patients are likely to experience proteinuria, decreased renal function, and a progressive drop in eGFR.

3. **Glomerulonephritis:** This occurs due to inflammation of the glomeruli, or filtering units of the kidney, caused by infections, autoimmune disorders, or other systemic illnesses. The immune system targets the glomeruli, causing inflammation and deterioration of kidney function. Patients are likely to experience proteinuria, hematuria (blood in the urine), and impaired kidney function as symptoms.

4. **PKD (Polycystic Kidney Disease):** This is a genetic condition that results in the formation of many cysts in the kidneys. These cysts form in the kidneys, causing swelling and eventually impairing kidney function. Patients should watch out for Symptoms like; Enlarged kidneys, hypertension, hematuria, and eventually kidney failure.

5. **Nephrotic Syndrome:** This happens when infections, medicines, or autoimmune reactions cause inflammation of the renal tubules and surrounding tissues. These inflammation causes tubule damage, affecting kidney function and urine concentration. Patients are likely to observe decreased urine concentration, electrolyte abnormalities, and reduced renal function.

6. **The Alport Syndrome:** This erupts as a result of a genetic condition that affects collagen in the glomeruli of the kidney and other organs. Abnormal collagen production damages the glomeruli, causing kidney damage and failure. Patients are likely to experience hematuria, hearing loss, and visual issues. Frequently develops to ESKD.

7. **CAKUT (Congenital Anomalies of the Kidney and Urinary Tract):** This is caused by developmental kidney or urinary tract abnormalities present at birth. Kidney function and urine flow are affected by malformations or structural problems. Symptoms vary based on the specific aberration, but can result in impaired kidney function.

8. **Other uncommon causes include:** These include inherited metabolic problems, kidney malignancies, kidney infections (such as HIV-associated nephropathy), and drug-induced kidney injury.

Risk Factors of Chronic Kidney Disease Women Should Look Out For

A number of risk factors can predispose women to Stage 3 chronic kidney disease (CKD), these factors are:

1. **Diabetes:** Women who have diabetes, particularly type 1 or type 2 diabetes, are at a higher risk of developing CKD. Elevated blood sugar levels can damage the kidneys over time, resulting to CKD.

2. **Hypertension (High Blood Pressure):** In women, chronic high blood pressure is a major risk factor for CKD. Uncontrolled hypertension can damage kidney blood vessels, limiting their function.

3. **Age:** Both men and women are at risk for CKD as they get older. Women's chance of having CKD rises with age, especially after the age of 50.

4. **Family History:** Having a family history of kidney disease, often known as CKD, can raise the risk in women. Kidney difficulties may be caused by genetic predispositions or inherited disorders.

5. **Obesity:** Being overweight or obese increases the likelihood of having CKD. Obesity adds to diabetes and hypertension, two major risk factors for kidney disease.

6. **Smoking:** This is a risk factor for a variety of health disorders, including CKD. Women who smoke have a higher chance of acquiring kidney disease than nonsmokers.

7. **Autoimmune illnesses:** Lupus (systemic lupus erythematosus) and other autoimmune illnesses are more common in women and can cause inflammation and damage to the kidneys.

8. **Urinary Tract Infections (UTIs):** If left untreated or becomes chronic, frequent or recurring urinary tract infections, which are more common in women, can cause kidney damage.

9. **Pregnancy-Related Complications:** Some pregnancy complications, such as preeclampsia (high blood pressure during pregnancy), can raise the risk of developing CKD later in life.

10. **Medication usage:** Certain medications, particularly long-term usage of nonsteroidal anti-inflammatory drugs (NSAIDs), can potentially cause kidney damage, particularly when used in high dosages or for long periods of time.

11. **Other illnesses:** Chronic illnesses such as heart disease, vascular disorders, and metabolic syndrome can all raise a woman's risk of CKD.

Early Symptoms of Chronic Kidney Disease in Women

Chronic Kidney Disease (CKD) Stage 3 frequently proceeds silently, with no obvious symptoms in the early stages. However, as kidney function deteriorates more, a variety of signs and symptoms may emerge, signaling the need for medical intervention. Here is a comprehensive list of symptoms related with CKD Stage 3:

1. **Weakness and fatigue:** Tiredness, weakness, or a lack of energy, even after enough rest, is a common symptom when kidney function declines and anemia develops.

2. **Edema (swelling):** Fluid accumulation in the body causes swelling, which is most typically seen in the legs, ankles, feet, or around the eyes due to inadequate fluid management by the kidneys.

3. **Urination Changes:** Urination patterns may change, such as increased frequency or decreased volume, foamy or bubbling urine (indicating proteinuria), and difficulty urinating.

4. **Retention of Fluid:** Fluid buildup as a result of impaired kidney function can produce puffiness, especially around the eyes, as well as shortness of breath due to fluid accumulating in the lungs.

5. **Hypertension (high blood pressure):** Hypertension or increased blood pressure may develop or worsen as a result of CKD, and is sometimes one of the first symptoms of renal impairment.

6. **Proteinuria:** Proteinuria (the presence of protein in the urine) is an indication of kidney injury. It may not cause obvious symptoms at first, but it can be discovered with urine tests.

7. **Anemia:** A decrease in erythropoietin production, a hormone generated by the kidneys, leads to a decrease in red blood cell synthesis, leading in anemia. Tiredness, weakness, and pale skin are some of the signs.

8. **Vomiting and nausea:** A accumulation of waste materials in the blood as a result of reduced kidney function may cause gastrointestinal symptoms such as nausea, vomiting, or loss of appetite.

9. **Problems with Bone Health:** Weakened bones, bone pain, or fractures may occur as a result of changes in mineral and bone metabolism induced by impaired renal function.

10. **Pruritus (itching):** A buildup of waste products in the blood, such as urea, can cause acute itching of the skin, but the cause may not be immediately apparent.

11. **Cognitive Shifts:** As CKD advances, the buildup of toxins in the body might cause cognitive impairment, trouble concentrating, or memory issues.

12. **Cardiovascular Problems:** Because of the influence on blood vessel health and the cardiovascular system, CKD raises the risk of cardiovascular disorders such as heart disease, heart attacks, and stroke.

Diagnosis and Monitoring of CKD Stage 3 in Women

Diagnosis and monitoring of chronic kidney disease (CKD) Stage 3 in women entail a variety of tests and examinations designed to measure kidney function, identify potential problems, and guide treatment options. Below are some vital things to know about diagnosis and what you should be expecting when you meet your doctor;

1. Medical History and Physical Examination:

To identify symptoms and risk factors associated with CKD, healthcare providers analyze the patient's medical history, family history, and do a physical exam.

2. **Blood Tests:** A sample of blood is carefully collected using a syringe and it's evaluated for the following below:

- **Serum creatinine test:** This estimates Glomerular Filtration Rate (eGFR) by measuring the waste product creatinine in the blood.

- **Blood urea nitrogen (BUN) test:** This evaluates how well the kidneys filter waste.

3. **Urine Tests:** This test is performed by getting a sample of urine from the woman. Below are what are evaluated during this test.

- **Urinalysis:** Detects urine abnormalities such as proteinuria, hematuria, and other indicators of kidney disease.

- **Urine albumin-to-creatinine ratio (UACR):** Indicates kidney impairment by measuring the amount of protein (albumin) in the urine.

4. **Imaging Studies:** Kidney ultrasound or CT scan; determines kidney size and structure, as well as any abnormalities or obstructions.

5. **eGFR Calculation:** eGFR is calculated to define the stage of CKD using formulas based on serum creatinine levels, age, gender, and race.

Monitoring

1. **Regular Follow-Up Visits:** Patients are advised to prioritize their appointments with healthcare providers, such as nephrologists or primary care physicians, to monitor and evaluate kidney function and overall health.

2. **Blood Pressure Monitoring:** A regular blood pressure monitoring and control are critical for managing and preventing future kidney injury in patients. Hence patients should ensure that their blood pressures are always in check.

3. **Blood and Urine Tests:** Patients should ensure they go for periodic blood tests (creatinine, BUN) and urine tests (urinalysis, UACR) to evaluate kidney function, proteinuria, and other kidney health indicators.

4. **eGFR Monitoring:** eGFR should be measured on a regular basis to evaluate changes in renal function and the course of CKD.

5. **Controlling consequences:** This includes monitoring and controlling CKD-related consequences such as anemia, bone disease, electrolyte abnormalities, and cardiovascular difficulties.

6. **Medication Review:** Monitoring medications, altering dosages, or changing prescriptions as needed to reduce the risk of kidney-related adverse effects or drug interactions.

7. **Dietary Management:** Patients should ensure they work closely with nutritionists to provide tailored dietary recommendations, with an emphasis on low-potassium, low-phosphorus, and kidney-friendly diet regimens.

8. **Lifestyle Counseling:** Patients should adopt some lifestyle changes such as exercise, smoking cessation, weight management, and stress management to support overall kidney health.

How Women Can Adopt Preventive Measures of CKD Stage 3

Adopting these preventative steps and incorporating healthy behaviors into everyday life can minimize the chance of development to CKD Stage 3 or slow the disease's course. Individualized assistance from healthcare specialists is critical in properly adopting these measures and customizing them to specific health needs and situations.

1. **Maintain Blood Sugar Levels (In Diabetes):** Maintaining appropriate blood sugar levels through medication, food, exercise, and regular monitoring is critical for diabetics to avoid kidney injury.

2. **Control High Blood Pressure:** Maintaining a healthy blood pressure (typically less than 130/80 mmHg) helps prevent additional kidney injury. Changes in lifestyle, drugs, and regular blood pressure monitoring are all necessary.

3. **Follow a Kidney-Friendly Diet:** A healthy diet rich in fruits, vegetables, whole grains, and lean meats that is low in salt, saturated fats, and processed foods can help regulate blood pressure and lessen the stress on the kidneys.

4. **Monitor Protein consumption:** Limiting protein consumption, particularly for patients with kidney illness, can reduce the stress on the kidneys. For personalized advice, speak with a healthcare physician or a dietician.

5. **Stay Hydrated:** Drinking enough of water aids with kidney function. Individuals with specific renal diseases, on the other hand, may need to check their fluid intake as directed by a healthcare practitioner.

6. **Avoid Nephrotoxic drugs:** Avoid drugs that can injure the kidneys, such as certain medications (NSAIDs, antibiotics), excessive painkiller usage, and exposure to certain poisons or chemicals.

7. **Regular Exercise:** Regular physical exercise helps manage blood pressure, control weight, and enhance general health, all of which promote kidney health indirectly.

8. **Quit Smoking:** Smoking can aggravate kidney disease and cardiovascular disease. Quitting smoking can reduce the risk of kidney injury and its effects considerably.

9. **Monitor Kidney Function:** Regular health screenings, including blood tests to assess kidney function (e.g., eGFR, creatinine levels) and urine tests for proteinuria, aid in early identification and intervention.

10. **Manage Underlying problems:** Proper management and control of underlying problems such as diabetes, hypertension, autoimmune diseases, and other health difficulties are critical in preventing additional kidney damage.

11 **Limit your alcohol consumption:** Moderation in alcohol use benefits general health and renal function. Excessive alcohol use can strain the kidneys and aggravate renal disease.

12. **Collaborate with Healthcare Providers:** Regular visits to healthcare providers, particularly nephrologists or primary care physicians, aid in kidney health monitoring, medication management, and receiving individualized kidney disease management advice.

Adopting a Kidney-Friendly Diet

Adopting a kidney-friendly diet is critical in controlling chronic kidney disease (CKD) and preventing future renal function degradation. Below are the benefits of adopting a kidney-friendly diet:

1. **Stress Reduction for the Kidneys:** A kidney-friendly diet seeks to lessen the workload on the kidneys by limiting the intake of substances that can strain the kidneys. This slows CKD progression and lowers complications.

2. **Blood Pressure Control:** A low-sodium diet aids with blood pressure control. Because high blood pressure can cause further kidney damage, lowering sodium consumption is critical in controlling and avoiding hypertension.

3. **Reduce Protein Intake:** Protein restriction reduces the stress on the kidneys because excessive protein metabolism produces waste products that the kidneys struggle to filter. This aids in the control of urea levels in the blood.

4. **Phosphorus and potassium control:** The kidneys control the levels of phosphorus and potassium in the blood. These levels can become unbalanced in CKD. A kidney-friendly diet helps restrict the intake of phosphorus and potassium-rich foods, minimizing strain on the kidneys.

5. **Fluid Intake Management:** Controlling fluid intake becomes critical for people with severe CKD. A kidney-friendly diet advises on how to regulate fluid consumption to avoid fluid retention and consequences such as edema or shortness of breath.

6. **Bone Health:** CKD can have an influence on bone health due to mineral imbalances. A kidney-friendly diet promotes optimal calcium and phosphorus balance, sustaining bone health and preventing CKD-related bone disorders.

7. **Enhancing Nutritional Status:** Regardless of dietary restrictions, a kidney-friendly diet stresses getting enough critical nutrients, vitamins, and minerals for overall health. It ensures that people with CKD get enough nourishment while dealing with kidney-related constraints.

8. **Promoting Overall Health:** A kidney-friendly diet not only improves renal function but also promotes overall

health by encouraging the consumption of fruits and vegetables, whole grains, and lean proteins, all of which contribute to heart health, weight control, and general well-being.

9. **Delaying the Need for Dialysis or Kidney Transplantation:** Adhering to a kidney-friendly diet, in conjunction with other lifestyle changes and adequate medical management, can help slow the progression of CKD, delaying the need for dialysis or kidney transplantation.

10 **Personalized Approach:** A kidney-friendly diet is adapted to individual needs, taking into account CKD stage, nutritional demands, other health issues, and personal preferences. For personalized nutritional suggestions, seek the advice of a licensed nutritionist or healthcare practitioner. In the pages ahead, we will delve into meal planning; a vital tool in combating CKD.

Meal Planning

Meal planning is a proactive nutrition approach that encourages healthy eating habits, saves time and money, decreases stress, and allows for a varied and balanced diet. It's a must-have for anyone looking to improve their overall health and well-being via attentive and deliberate meal planning.

Strategies of Meal Planning

1. **Strategic Preparation:** Meal planning entails careful consideration and preparation of meals for a set period of time, usually a week or more. It includes determining what to eat, making grocery lists, and planning meals ahead of time.

2. **A Variety of Meals:** It enables the creation of a wide range of balanced, nutritious meals that incorporate various food

groups, flavors, and textures to match dietary needs and preferences.

3. **Time and Resource Management:** Meal planning saves time and money by lowering the number of grocery shopping, eliminating food waste, and streamlining meal preparation on busy days.

Advantages of Meal Planning

1. **Improved Eating Habits:** Meal planning makes it easier to include nutritious meals in appropriate portions, assisting persons in maintaining a well-balanced diet with necessary nutrients, vitamins, and minerals.

2. **Reduces Time:** Dinner planning saves time by decreasing the need for daily food decisions and streamlining grocery shopping and dinner preparation.

3. **Affordability:** It can help with budgeting by lowering impulse purchases and food waste. Planning meals around goods that are on sale or in season might help you save money.

4. **Portion Control and Weight Control:** Meal planning promotes portion control by pre-determining portion sizes and managing ingredients, which aids with weight management goals.

5. **Reduces Stress:** Knowing what meals to prepare ahead of time alleviates the stress associated with last-minute meal decisions and frantic cooking on busy days.

6. **Expanded Variety and Creativity:** Meal planning allows for greater creativity in meal selection and preparation, as well as the introduction of new recipes, cuisines, and flavors for a more diverse dining experience.

The Benefits of Meal Planning

1. **Nutrition and Health:** It ensures that people eat balanced meals, meeting their nutritional needs and avoiding the use of less nutritious options such as fast food or processed meals.

2. **Time Efficiency:** Meal planning saves time by combining grocery shopping and dinner preparation, making it easier to manage hectic schedules and cut cooking time in half.

3. **Consistency and Routine:** It aids in the establishment of a routine and consistent eating pattern, which promotes general health and wellness.

4. **Flexibility and Adaptability:** Meal planning allows you to meet dietary restrictions, preferences, or schedule changes without sacrificing nutritional quality.

5. **Empowerment and Control:** Taking charge of meal planning allows people to make healthier food choices, change their eating habits, and better manage their diet-related goals.

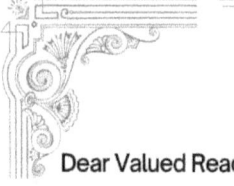
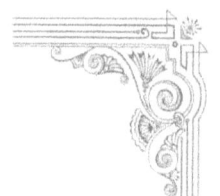

Dear Valued Reader,

Thank you for selecting our cookbook from among the many available. Your decision to live a healthy lifestyle with the help of our book means everything to us. We welcome you to share your thoughts on the website by leaving a polite review. Your feedback supports our journey, and we are grateful. Let your words be the heartbeat of our collective dedication to happiness. We also humbly request that you visit and follow our author page; by doing so, you will be exposed to a plethora of other publications by this author.

With appreciation,

DR. LUNA O. RICHARDS

Part Two

Making Quick and Easy Renal Friendly Recipes

I welcome you, my dear readers, to Part 2 of our book. In the previous chapter, we discussed a lot about kidney disease, its causes, diagnosis, preventive measures, and types of CKD.

All of the above was preparatory to this part of our book, because having to understand what you are up against gives you an edge to advance over that challenge.

This part of our book is intended not only for the palette but also for the vitality of the body and soul. In the pages that follow, we will delve into a world where health meets flavor, where nourishment goes beyond ordinary sustenance—a world designed exclusively for women challenged with the complexities of chronic kidney disease (CKD) stage 3.

Prepare to go on a revolutionary voyage of nutrition, where each cuisine is a step toward wellbeing and each ingredient has been carefully selected for your health and wellness. But, before we go on this taste adventure, I will be providing you with a detailed grocery shopping list adapted for CKD, which I used in making these recipes time after time. Enjoy!

Grocery Shopping List

This comprehensive shopping list covers the ingredients needed for the listed recipes while ensuring compliance with a kidney-friendly, low-potassium, and phosphorus-conscious diet. Adjust quantities based on serving sizes and personal preferences. Planning and shopping with this list can streamline the grocery shopping process, helping individuals with CKD Stage 3 spend less time in the store while ensuring they have everything they need to prepare their kidney-friendly meals.

Fruits:

- Blueberries

- Strawberries

- Raspberries

- Apples

- Bananas

- Lemons

- Watermelon

- Avocado

Vegetables:

- Spinach

- Bell Peppers (red, green, yellow)

- Zucchini

- Cauliflower

- Tomatoes

- Eggplant

- Cucumbers

- Mushrooms

- Kale

Grains and Legumes:

- Quinoa

- Lentils

- Chickpeas

- Black Beans

- Brown Rice

- Almond Flour

Protein Sources:

- Tofu

- Tempeh

- Chia Seeds

Dairy Alternatives:

- Almond Milk

- Coconut Milk

Herbs and Spices:

- Cinnamon

- Ginger

- Basil

- Oregano

- Thyme

- Mint

- Turmeric

- Garlic

- Onion

- Black Pepper

Condiments and Others:

- Olive Oil

- Low-sodium Vegetable Broth

- Low-sodium Soy Sauce

- Tahini

- Apple Cider Vinegar

- Baking Powder

- Baking Soda

Nuts and Seeds:

- Almonds

- Flaxseeds

Snacks:

- Chickpea Snacks

- Low-Potassium Chips

Frozen Section:

- Frozen Berries (Blueberries, Strawberries)

- Frozen Mixed Vegetables

Beverages:

- Herbal Teas (Chamomile, Peppermint)

- Fresh Apples for Juice

- Ingredients for Smoothies (Cucumber, Spinach)

Dessert:

- Unsweetened Coconut Milk (for making coconut milk ice cream)

- Ingredients for Baked Apples (such as cinnamon)

Miscellaneous:

- Low-Potassium Baking Ingredients (if necessary)

- Low-Potassium Snack Options (as desired)

Tips for Effective Grocery Shopping

Following these tips can streamline the grocery shopping process, help you make informed choices, and ensure you have the necessary ingredients for kidney-friendly meals while managing CKD Stage 3 successfully. Always contact a healthcare professional or dietitian for personalized dietary guidance and recommendations based on individual health needs.

1. **Plan Ahead:** Make a list of needed items based on planned meals to avoid impulse buying and ensure you have all the necessary materials.

2. **Stick to the List**: Focus on purchasing items from your prepared list to avoid overspending and minimize buying unnecessary items.

3. **Read Labels:** Check nutrition labels for potassium and phosphorus content, opting for low-potassium and low-phosphorus options when possible.

4. **Shop the Perimeter:** Most fresh produce, dairy alternatives, and low-phosphorus protein sources are usually located around the store's perimeter. Concentrate on these sections for healthier choices.

5. **Buy Seasonal Produce:** Seasonal fruits and veggies are often fresher, more flavorful, and may be more affordable. Consider buying these choices to diversify your meals.

6. **Choose Low-Potassium Alternatives:** Select low-potassium fruits and vegetables like apples, berries, cucumbers, and cauliflower instead of high-potassium choices like bananas or potatoes.

7. **Opt for Low-Phosphorus Foods:** Look for low-phosphorus grains, legumes, and protein sources such as quinoa, brown rice, lentils, and tofu to control phosphorus intake.

8. **Stock Up on Staples:** Purchase non-perishable staples like herbs, spices, low-sodium broths, oils, and nuts/seeds to have important ingredients on hand for meal preparation.

9. **Check for Sales and Discounts:** Look for sales or discounts on items you frequently use but ensure they fit with your dietary restrictions and needs.

10. **Consider Frozen or Canned Options:** Frozen or canned fruits and veggies can be good alternatives when fresh options are not available. Look for no-salt-added or low-sodium options.

11. **Avoid Highly Processed Foods:** Limit purchases of processed and packaged foods that often contain high amounts of sodium, phosphorus additives, and preservatives.

12. **Plan for Snacks and Beverages**: Include low-potassium snacks and beverages on your list, such as unsalted nuts, chickpea snacks, herbal teas, and fresh fruits perfect for juicing.

13. **Use Reusable Bags and Stay Organized**: Bring reusable bags to reduce plastic waste and keep things organized during checkout and transport.

14. **Shop During Off-Peak Hours:** Avoid peak shopping times to lower crowds and make shopping more efficient and less stressful.

15. **Stay Hydrated:** Drink water before shopping to stay hydrated, focused, and less likely to make spontaneous purchases.

After a successful shopping section, we will now focus on preparing these food stuffs in the healthiest way possible. In the coming pages of our book, we will delve into how you can make these low sodium, low potassium, low phosphorus recipes with ease. ***Happy cooking ahead!***

Bravo!!!

If you have read our book to this point, it shows you really care about your kidney health and wellness, we hope your awareness towards kidney disease have appreciated positively.

As you advance into the cookbook portion of our book, we will dwell on how to make these renal friendly breakfasts, lunch, desserts, beverages and snacks without sacrificing taste and time.

We trust you are enjoying your read, to serve you better we sincerely ask you to drop your kind review about using this book in the website, as this will help us know what interests you, and model our subsequent books to meet your needs.

You can kindly check out some other books on kidney disease by this author. Click the respective book links below to get a copy of these books, or scan the QR Codes to gain access.

Chronic Kidney Disease Stage 3 Cookbook for Men

Kidney Disease Diet Stage 3 Cookbook

Chronic Kidney Disease Stage 3 Cookbook for Beginners

 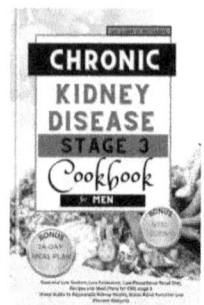

Scan the Code to get the Chronic Kidney Disease Stage 3 Cookbook for Men

 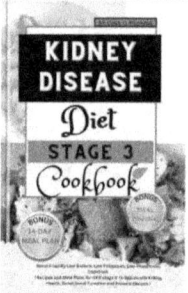

Scan the Code to get the Kidney Disease Stage 3 Cookbook

 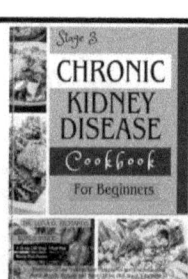

Scan the Code to get the Chronic Kidney Disease Stage 3 Cookbook for Beginners

 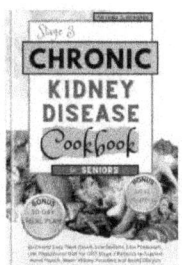

Scan the Code to get the Chronic Kidney Disease
Stage 3 Cookbook for Seniors

Breakfast Recipes

Recipe 1: *Quinoa Breakfast Bowl*

A wholesome and nutritious breakfast option, this Quinoa Breakfast Bowl offers a blend of protein, fiber, and essential nutrients to kickstart your day.

PREP TIME: 5 MINUTES

COOK TIME: 15 MINUTES

TOTAL TIME: 20 MINUTES

SERVINGS: 2

Ingredients:

- 1 cup quinoa, rinsed
- 2 cups almond milk (or any preferred milk)
- 1 tablespoon maple syrup (optional)
- 1/2 teaspoon ground cinnamon
- 1/4 teaspoon vanilla extract
- 1 cup mixed fresh berries (such as strawberries, blueberries, raspberries)

- Two tablespoons of chopped nuts (almonds, walnuts, or pecans)
- Fresh mint leaves, for garnish (optional)

Instructions:

1. In a saucepan, combine quinoa and almond milk. Bring to a boil over medium heat.

2. Reduce heat to low, cover, and simmer for 15 minutes or until quinoa is cooked and liquid is absorbed.

3. Stir in maple syrup (if using), ground cinnamon, and vanilla extract. Mix well.

4. Divide the cooked quinoa into serving bowls.

5. Top each bowl with mixed fresh berries and chopped nuts.

6. Decorate with fresh mint leaves, if desired.

7. Serve warm and enjoy this delightful Quinoa Breakfast Bowl!

Nutritional Value (per serving):

- Calories: 320 kcal
- Protein: 10g
- Fat: 8g
- Carbohydrates: 52g
- Fiber: 6g
- Sodium: 110mg
- Potassium: 370mg

Recipe 2: *Blueberry Chia Seed Pudding*

A delicious and nutritious make-ahead breakfast or snack, this Blueberry Chia Seed Pudding is rich in antioxidants, omega-3 fatty acids, and fiber.

PREP TIME: 5 MINUTES (plus chilling time)

COOK TIME: 0 MINUTES

TOTAL TIME: 4 HOURS (Chilling time)

SERVINGS: 2

Ingredients:

- 1 cup of unsweetened almond milk (or any preferred milk)
- 1/4 cup chia seeds
- One tablespoon of maple syrup (or sweetener of choice)
- 1/2 teaspoon vanilla extract
- 1/2 cup fresh blueberries
- 2 tablespoons chopped nuts (such as almonds or walnuts)
- Additional blueberries for topping (optional)

Instructions:

1. In a mixing bowl, combine almond milk, chia seeds, maple syrup, and vanilla extract. Stir well to combine.

2. Gently fold in fresh blueberries.

3. Cover the bowl and refrigerate for at least 4 hours or overnight, allowing the chia seeds to expand and create a pudding-like consistency.

4. Stir the mixture before serving to evenly distribute the chia seeds.

5. Divide the Blueberry Chia Seed Pudding into serving bowls.

6. Top with chopped nuts and additional fresh blueberries, if desired.

7. Serve chilled and savor this delightful and healthy pudding!

Nutritional Value (per serving):

- Calories: 210 kcal
- Protein: 6g
- Fat: 12g
- Carbohydrates: 22g
- Fiber: 12g
- Sodium: 80mg
- Potassium: 220mg

Recipe 3: *Vegetable Omelette with Spinach and Peppers*

A nutritious and flavorful breakfast choice, this Vegetable Omelette with Spinach and Peppers is packed with protein and essential nutrients to start your day right.

PREP TIME: 10 MINUTES

COOK TIME: 5 MINUTES

TOTAL TIME: 15 MINUTES

SERVINGS: 2

Ingredients:

- 4 large eggs
- Quarter cup of diced bell peppers (any color)
- 1/2 cup chopped fresh spinach leaves
- 1/4 cup diced onions
- 2 tablespoons chopped fresh parsley
- Salt and pepper, to taste
- 1 tablespoon olive oil

Instructions:

1. In a bowl, crack the eggs and beat them until well combined. Add diced bell peppers, chopped spinach, diced onions, parsley, and season with salt and pepper. Mix thoroughly.

2. Heat olive oil in a non-stick skillet over medium heat.

3. Pour the egg mixture into the skillet, spreading it evenly to cover the surface. Cook for 2-3 minutes or until the bottom is set.

4. Using a spatula, carefully lift the edges of the omelette and slightly tilt the skillet to allow uncooked eggs to flow underneath.

5. Once the omelette is mostly set but still slightly moist on top, fold it in half using the spatula.

6. Cook for another 1-2 minutes or until cooked through and golden on the outside.

7. Slide the omelette onto a plate and garnish with extra parsley, if desired.

8. Serve hot and enjoy this delightful Vegetable Omelette with Spinach and Peppers!

Nutritional Value (per serving):

- Calories: 180 kcal
- Protein: 12g
- Fat: 13g
- Carbohydrates: 4g
- Fiber: 1g
- Sodium: 150mg
- Potassium: 230mg

Recipe 4: *Almond Flour Pancakes with Berries*

A delicious and gluten-free breakfast treat, these Almond Flour Pancakes with Berries are light, fluffy, and bursting with fruity goodness.

PREP TIME: 10 MINUTES

COOK TIME: 10 MINUTES

TOTAL TIME: 20 MINUTES

SERVINGS: 2-3

Ingredients:

- 1 cup almond flour
- 2 large eggs
- 1/4 cup of unsweetened almond milk (or any preferred milk)
- 1 tablespoon maple syrup (optional)
- 1/2 teaspoon baking powder
- 1/2 teaspoon vanilla extract
- 1/2 cup fresh mixed berries (such as blueberries, strawberries)
- Coconut oil or butter for cooking

Instructions:

1. In a mixing bowl, whisk together almond flour, eggs, almond milk, maple syrup (if using), baking powder, and vanilla extract until a smooth batter forms.

2. Gently fold in the fresh mixed berries into the batter.

3. Heat a non-stick skillet or griddle over medium heat and lightly grease it with coconut oil or butter.

4. Pour a scoop of pancake batter onto the skillet to form pancakes of desired size.

5. Cook for 2-3 minutes on one side or until bubbles form on the surface.

6. Carefully flip the pancakes and cook for another 1-2 minutes or until golden brown and cooked through.

7. Repeat with the remaining batter, adding more oil or butter to the skillet as needed.

8. Stack the Almond Flour Pancakes on a plate, top with additional berries if desired, and serve warm.

9. Enjoy these delightful Almond Flour Pancakes with Berries for a delicious and wholesome breakfast!

Nutritional Value (per serving - 2 pancakes):

- Calories: 280 kcal

- Protein: 12g
- Fat: 22g
- Carbohydrates: 14g
- Fiber: 6g
- Sodium: 80mg
- Potassium: 180mg

Recipe 5: *Avocado Toast with Low-Potassium Toppings*

This Avocado Toast with Low-Potassium Toppings is a nutritious and flavorful breakfast or snack option, perfect for those with dietary restrictions.

PREP TIME: 5 MINUTES

COOK TIME: 5 MINUTES

TOTAL TIME: 10 MINUTES

SERVINGS: 2

Ingredients:

- 2 slices whole-grain bread (low-sodium if available)

- 1 ripe avocado, peeled and pitted
- 1 tablespoon lemon juice
- Low-potassium toppings options:
- Diced cucumber
- Sliced radishes
- Alfalfa sprouts
- Fresh basil leaves
- Sesame seeds (optional)
- Salt and pepper, to taste

Instructions:

1. Toast the slices of whole-grain bread until they reach desired crispness.

2. In a bowl, mash the ripe avocado with a fork. Add lemon juice, salt, and pepper. Mix until well combined.

3. Evenly spread the mashed avocado onto the toasted bread slices.

4. Top the avocado toast with low-potassium toppings such as diced cucumber, sliced radishes, alfalfa sprouts, fresh basil leaves, or sprinkle with sesame seeds if desired.

5. Add with a pinch of salt and pepper to taste.

6. Serve the Avocado Toast with Low-Potassium Toppings immediately and enjoy this delicious and kidney-friendly dish!

Nutritional Value (per serving - 1 slice):

- Calories: 180 kcal
- Protein: 4g
- Fat: 11g
- Carbohydrates: 18g
- Fiber: 6g
- Sodium: 120mg
- Potassium: 360mg

Lunch Recipes

Recipe 1: *Lentil and Vegetable Soup*

A hearty and nourishing soup, this Lentil and Vegetable Soup is loaded with fiber, plant-based protein, and wholesome ingredients for a satisfying meal.

PREP TIME: 15 MINUTES

COOK TIME: 40 MINUTES

TOTAL TIME: 55 MINUTES

SERVINGS: 4-6

Ingredients:

- 1 cup of dried green or brown lentils, rinsed
- 6 cups low-sodium vegetable broth
- 1 onion, finely chopped
- 2 carrots, diced
- 2 celery stalks, diced

- 2 cloves garlic, minced
- 1 can (14 oz) diced tomatoes (low-sodium if available)
- 1 teaspoon ground cumin
- 1 teaspoon paprika
- 1/2 teaspoon dried thyme
- Salt and pepper, to taste
- Fresh parsley for garnish (optional)

Instructions:

1. In a large pot, combine the rinsed lentils and vegetable broth. Over medium-high heat, boil the vegetable broth and rinsed lentils, then reduce heat to low and simmer for 20 minutes.

2. In a separate skillet, heat a bit of olive oil over medium heat. Pour in the chopped onion, carrots, celery, and minced garlic. Fry for 5-6 minutes until vegetables begin to soften.

3. Add the sautéed vegetables, diced tomatoes (with juices), ground cumin, paprika, dried thyme, salt, and pepper to the pot with lentils. Stir to combine.

4. Continue simmering the soup for an additional 15-20 minutes or until lentils and vegetables are tender.

5. Adjust seasoning to taste and add more broth if desired for a thinner consistency.

6. Ladle the Lentil and Vegetable Soup into bowls, garnish with fresh parsley if desired, and serve hot.

7. Enjoy this comforting Lentil and Vegetable Soup as a wholesome and kidney-friendly meal!

Nutritional Value (per serving - estimated for 1/6 of the recipe):

- Calories: 200 kcal
- Protein: 12g
- Fat: 1g
- Carbohydrates: 36g
- Fiber: 11g

- Sodium: 220mg
- Potassium: 560mg

Recipe 2: *Chickpea Salad Wraps*

These Chickpea Salad Wraps are a delightful, protein-packed option for a satisfying and flavorful meal or snack.

PREP TIME: 15 MINUTES

COOK TIME: 0 MINUTES

TOTAL TIME: 15 MINUTES

SERVINGS: 2-4

Ingredients:

- One can (15 oz) of chickpeas, drained and rinsed
- 1/4 cup diced red bell pepper
- 1/4 cup diced cucumber
- 2 tablespoons diced red onion
- 2 tablespoons of chopped fresh parsley or cilantro
- 2 tablespoons lemon juice

- 2 tablespoons olive oil
- Salt and pepper, to taste
- Lettuce leaves or whole-grain wraps
- Optional add-ins: diced tomatoes, avocado slices

Instructions:

1. In a mixing bowl, add the drained and rinsed chickpeas. Use a fork or potato masher to lightly mash some of the chickpeas, leaving some whole for texture.

2. Add diced red bell pepper, cucumber, red onion, chopped parsley or cilantro, lemon juice, olive oil, salt, and pepper to the bowl with the chickpeas. Mix well to combine.

3. Place a spoonful of the chickpea salad onto lettuce leaves or whole-grain wraps.

4. Add optional ingredients like diced tomatoes or avocado slices if desired.

5. Roll the lettuce leaves or wraps to form Chickpea Salad Wraps.

6. Serve these delicious wraps immediately or refrigerate for a refreshing and satisfying meal or snack!

Nutritional Value (per serving - estimated for 1 wrap):

- Calories: 210 kcal
- Protein: 8g
- Fat: 10g
- Carbohydrates: 25g
- Fiber: 7g
- Sodium: 180mg
- Potassium: 290mg

Recipe 3: *Zucchini Noodles with Pesto Sauce*

This Zucchini Noodles with Pesto Sauce dish offers a light and flavorful alternative to traditional pasta, perfect for a low-carb and nutrient-rich meal.

PREP TIME: 15 MINUTES

COOK TIME: 5 MINUTES

TOTAL TIME: 20 MINUTES

SERVINGS: 2-3

Ingredients:

- 4 medium-sized zucchinis
- 1/2 cup of basil pesto sauce (store-bought or homemade)
- 1 tablespoon olive oil
- Cherry tomatoes, halved (for garnish, optional)
- Pine nuts (for garnish, optional)
- Fresh basil leaves (for garnish, optional)
- Salt and pepper, to taste

Instructions:

1. Wash the zucchinis and trim the ends. Create a zucchini noodles ("zoodles") with a spiralizer or a vegetable peeler and set aside.

2. Heat up the olive oil over medium heat in a large skillet. Add the zucchini noodles to the skillet and sauté for 2-3 minutes or until slightly softened. Be cautious not to overcook; zoodles should remain slightly firm.

3. Transfer the sautéed zucchini noodles to a mixing bowl.

4. Add basil pesto sauce to the zucchini noodles and toss until the noodles are evenly coated.

5. Divide the Zucchini Noodles with Pesto Sauce into serving bowls.

6. Garnish with halved cherry tomatoes, pine nuts, and fresh basil leaves if desired.

7. Serve this delightful dish immediately as a light and flavorful alternative to pasta!

Nutritional Value (per serving - estimated for 1/3 of the recipe):

- Calories: 180 kcal
- Protein: 5g
- Fat: 15g

- Carbohydrates: 8g
- Fiber: 3g
- Sodium: 280mg
- Potassium: 600mg

Recipe 4: *Black Bean and Vegetable Burrito Bowl*

This Black Bean and Vegetable Burrito Bowl is a vibrant and nutritious dish, combining flavors and textures for a satisfying meal.

PREP TIME: 15 MINUTES

COOK TIME: 15 MINUTES

TOTAL TIME: 30 MINUTES

SERVINGS: 2-3

Ingredients:

- 1 cup cooked brown rice
- One can (15 oz) of black beans, drained and rinsed
- 1 tablespoon olive oil

- 1 red bell pepper, diced
- 1 yellow bell pepper, diced
- 1 small zucchini, diced
- One cup of corn kernels should be fresh or frozen.
- 1 teaspoon ground cumin
- 1 teaspoon chili powder
- Salt and pepper, to taste
- Toppings (optional):
- Sliced avocado
- Diced tomatoes
- Chopped fresh cilantro
- Lime wedges
- Salsa or hot sauce

Instructions:

1. Heat olive oil over medium heat (in a skillet). Add diced red and yellow bell peppers, zucchini, and corn kernels. Until vegetables are tender, fry for five to six minutes.

2. Add cooked black beans to the skillet along with ground cumin, chili powder, salt, and pepper. Stir to combine and cook for an additional 2-3 minutes.

3. Divide the cooked brown rice into serving bowls.

4. Spoon the black bean and vegetable mixture over the rice in each bowl.

5. Add optional toppings like sliced avocado, diced tomatoes, chopped fresh cilantro, and a squeeze of lime juice or salsa.

6. Serve this delicious Black Bean and Vegetable Burrito Bowl as a colorful and nutritious meal!

Nutritional Value (per serving - estimated for 1/3 of the recipe):

- Calories: 350 kcal
- Protein: 13g
- Fat: 7g
- Carbohydrates: 63g
- Fiber: 13g

- Sodium: 490mg
- Potassium: 810mg

Recipe 5: *Mushroom and Spinach Quinoa Salad*

This Mushroom and Spinach Quinoa Salad is a delightful blend of earthy flavors and nutritional goodness, perfect for a satisfying meal or side dish.

PREP TIME: 10 MINUTES

COOK TIME: 20 MINUTES

TOTAL TIME: 30 MINUTES

SERVINGS: 4

Ingredients:

- 1 cup quinoa, rinsed
- Two cups of low-sodium vegetable broth (or water)
- 1 tablespoon olive oil
- 8 oz mushrooms, sliced

- 2 cloves garlic, minced
- 4 cups fresh spinach leaves
- 1/4 cup chopped fresh parsley
- 2 tablespoons lemon juice
- Salt and pepper, to taste
- Optional add-ins:
- Cherry tomatoes, halved
- Sliced cucumber
- Crumbled feta cheese

Instructions:

1. In a saucepan, Bring the vegetable broth to a boil in a sauce pan. Add rinsed quinoa, reduce heat to low, cover, and simmer for 15-20 minutes or until quinoa is cooked and liquid is absorbed. Let it cool.

2. Heat olive oil over medium heat in a skillet. Add sliced mushrooms and minced garlic. Sauté for 5-6 minutes until mushrooms are tender and golden.

3. Add fresh spinach leaves to the skillet and cook for an additional 2-3 minutes until wilted.

4. In a large mixing bowl, combine cooked quinoa, sautéed mushrooms and spinach, chopped parsley, lemon juice, salt, and pepper. Toss gently to mix all ingredients.

5. Add optional add-ins like cherry tomatoes, sliced cucumber, or crumbled feta cheese if desired.

6. Serve this delightful Mushroom and Spinach Quinoa Salad as a nutritious and flavorful dish!

Nutritional Value (per serving - estimated for 1/4 of the recipe):

- Calories: 220 kcal
- Protein: 8g
- Fat: 6g
- Carbohydrates: 35g
- Fiber: 5g
- Sodium: 20mg
- Potassium: 500mg

Dinner Recipes

Recipe 1: *Baked Herb-Crusted Tofu with Steamed Vegetables*

This Baked Herb-Crusted Tofu with Steamed Vegetables is a flavorful and wholesome dish, packed with protein and nutritious veggies.

PREP TIME: 15 MINUTES

COOK TIME: 25 MINUTES

TOTAL TIME: 40 MINUTES

SERVINGS: 2-3

Ingredients:

- One block of (14 oz) extra-firm tofu, pressed and drained
- 2 tablespoons olive oil

- 2 tablespoons finely chopped fresh herbs (such as rosemary, thyme, parsley)
- 1/4 cup of breadcrumbs (use gluten-free if desired)
- Salt and pepper, to taste
- Assorted vegetables for steaming (broccoli, carrots, cauliflower, etc.)

Instructions:

1. Preheat the oven to 400°F (200°C).

2. Cut the pressed tofu into cubes or rectangular pieces.

3. In a bowl, mix olive oil, finely chopped fresh herbs, breadcrumbs, salt, and pepper.

4. Coat each tofu piece evenly with the herb and breadcrumb mixture.

5. Place the coated tofu pieces on a lined baking sheet.

6. Bake in the preheated oven for 20-25 minutes or until the tofu turns golden brown and crisp on the outside.

7. While the tofu is baking, steam the assorted vegetables until they are tender yet slightly crisp.

8. Once done, serve the Baked Herb-Crusted Tofu alongside steamed vegetables for a delightful and nutritious meal!

Nutritional Value (per serving - estimated for 1/3 of the recipe):

- Calories: 280 kcal
- Protein: 16g
- Fat: 17g
- Carbohydrates: 18g
- Fiber: 4g
- Sodium: 200mg
- Potassium: 470mg

Recipe 2: *Cauliflower Rice Stir-Fry with Tofu or Tempeh*

This Cauliflower Rice Stir-Fry with Tofu or Tempeh is a delicious, low-carb alternative to traditional rice, packed with veggies and plant-based protein.

PREP TIME: 15 MINUTES

COOK TIME: 15 MINUTES

TOTAL TIME: 30 MINUTES

SERVINGS: 2-3

Ingredients:

- 1 block (14 oz) tofu or tempeh, cubed
- 1 head cauliflower, grated into "rice" or store-bought cauliflower rice
- Two tablespoons of low-sodium soy sauce or tamari
- 1 tablespoon sesame oil
- 2 cloves garlic, minced
- 1 teaspoon grated ginger
- Assorted vegetables like bell peppers, broccoli, carrots, snap peas, etc.
- Green onions, chopped (for garnish)
- Sesame seeds (for garnish, optional)

Instructions:

1. Heat a non-stick skillet or wok over medium heat. Add cubed tofu or tempeh and cook until golden brown on all sides. Set aside.

2. In the same skillet, heat sesame oil over medium heat. Add minced garlic and grated ginger. Sauté for 1 minute until fragrant.

3. Add assorted vegetables to the skillet and stir-fry for 3-4 minutes until they begin to soften.

4. Push the vegetables to one side of the skillet and add cauliflower rice to the empty side.

5. Cook the cauliflower rice for 3-4 minutes, stirring occasionally, until it starts to soften.

6. Mix the cauliflower rice with the cooked vegetables in the skillet. Add low-sodium soy sauce or tamari and stir to combine.

7. Add the cooked tofu or tempeh back into the skillet and toss everything together until heated through.

8. Garnish with chopped green onions and sesame seeds if desired.

9. Serve this flavorful Cauliflower Rice Stir-Fry with Tofu or Tempeh as a satisfying and wholesome dish!

Nutritional Value (per serving - estimated for 1/3 of the recipe):

- Calories: 250 kcal
- Protein: 18g
- Fat: 12g
- Carbohydrates: 20g
- Fiber: 8g
- Sodium: 380mg
- Potassium: 780mg

Recipe 3: *Eggplant and Tomato Casserole*

This Eggplant and Tomato Casserole is a delightful Mediterranean-inspired dish, combining the flavors of eggplant, tomatoes, and aromatic herbs for a comforting meal.

PREP TIME: 20 MINUTES

COOK TIME: 45 MINUTES

TOTAL TIME: 1 HOUR 5 MINUTES

SERVINGS: 4-6

Ingredients:

- 2 medium-sized eggplants, thinly sliced
- 4 large tomatoes, thinly sliced
- 2 cloves garlic, minced
- 1/4 cup fresh basil leaves, chopped
- 1/4 cup fresh parsley, chopped
- 1/2 cup breadcrumbs (gluten-free if desired)
- 1/4 cup grated Parmesan cheese or nutritional yeast (for vegan option)
- 3 tablespoons olive oil
- Salt and pepper, to taste

Instructions:

1. Preheat the oven to 375°F (190°C). Lightly grease a baking dish with olive oil.

2. Arrange a layer of sliced eggplants at the bottom of the baking dish.

3. Layer sliced tomatoes on top of the eggplant. Sprinkle minced garlic, chopped basil, and parsley over the tomatoes.

4. Repeat layering with the remaining eggplant and tomatoes until all ingredients are used, finishing with a layer of tomatoes on top.

5. In a small bowl, mix breadcrumbs, grated Parmesan cheese or nutritional yeast, and olive oil until combined.

6. Sprinkle the breadcrumb mixture evenly over the top layer of tomatoes.

7. Cover the baking dish with foil and bake in the preheated oven for 30-35 minutes.

8. Remove the foil and continue baking for an additional 10-15 minutes or until the top is golden brown and bubbly.

9. Once done, let the Eggplant and Tomato Casserole cool slightly before serving.

10. Enjoy this delicious Mediterranean-inspired casserole as a flavorful and comforting meal!

Nutritional Value (per serving - estimated for 1/6 of the recipe):

- Calories: 120 kcal
- Protein: 4g
- Fat: 7g
- Carbohydrates: 14g
- Fiber: 7g
- Sodium: 90mg
- Potassium: 590mg

Recipe 4: *Vegan Lentil Shepherd's Pie*

This Vegan Lentil Shepherd's Pie is a hearty and nourishing dish, combining lentils, vegetables, and mashed potatoes for a comforting and satisfying meal.

PREP TIME: 20 MINUTES

COOK TIME: 45 MINUTES

TOTAL TIME: 1 HOUR 5 MINUTES

SERVINGS: 4-6

Ingredients:

- 4 large potatoes, peeled and cubed
- 2 tablespoons olive oil
- 1 onion, diced
- 2 carrots, diced
- 2 celery stalks, diced
- 2 cloves garlic, minced
- 1 cup cooked green or brown lentils
- 1 cup vegetable broth
- 2 tablespoons tomato paste
- 1 teaspoon dried thyme
- 1 teaspoon dried rosemary
- Salt and pepper, to taste
- Fresh parsley, chopped (for garnish)

Instructions:

1. Preheat the oven to 375°F (190°C).

2. Boil or steam the peeled and cubed potatoes until tender. Drain and mash them with a fork or potato masher, adding a bit of olive oil for creaminess. Set aside.

3. Heat up the olive oil over medium heat (in a skillet). Add diced onion, carrots, and celery. Until vegetables begin to soften, keep frying for five to six minutes.

4. Add minced garlic to the skillet and cook for an additional 1-2 minutes until fragrant.

5. Stir in cooked lentils, vegetable broth, tomato paste, dried thyme, dried rosemary, salt, and pepper. Cook gently for ten to twelve minutes until the mixture thickens.

6. Transfer the lentil and vegetable mixture to a baking dish.

7. Spread the mashed potatoes evenly over the lentil mixture in the baking dish.

8. Bake in the preheated oven for 25-30 minutes or until the top is golden brown and the filling is bubbling around the edges.

9. Once done, remove from the oven and let it cool slightly.

10. Garnish with fresh chopped parsley before serving this comforting Vegan Lentil Shepherd's Pie!

Nutritional Value (per serving - estimated for 1/6 of the recipe):

- Calories: 230 kcal
- Protein: 8g
- Fat: 6g
- Carbohydrates: 38g
- Fiber: 8g
- Sodium: 310mg
- Potassium: 820mg

Recipe 5: *Pasta Primavera with Kidney-Friendly Sauce*

This Pasta Primavera with Kidney-Friendly Sauce is a delightful dish combining colorful vegetables and a kidney-friendly sauce for a flavorful pasta experience.

PREP TIME: 15 MINUTES

COOK TIME: 20 MINUTES

TOTAL TIME: 35 MINUTES

SERVINGS: 4

Ingredients:

- 8 oz whole-grain pasta (choose low-phosphorus pasta if needed)
- 1 tablespoon olive oil
- 2 cloves garlic, minced
- 1 cup cherry tomatoes, halved
- 1 small zucchini, thinly sliced
- 1 cup broccoli florets
- 1 cup chopped spinach leaves
- Kidney-friendly sauce:
- 1 cup low-sodium vegetable broth
- 2 tablespoons tomato paste
- 1 teaspoon dried basil
- 1 teaspoon dried oregano

- Salt and pepper, to taste

Instructions:

1. Cook the pasta according to package instructions. Drain and set aside.

2. Heat up the olive oil over medium heat (in a large skillet). Add minced garlic and sauté for 1 minute until fragrant.

3. Add cherry tomatoes, zucchini, and broccoli florets to the skillet. Until the vegetables begin to soften, keep frying for five to six minutes.

4. In a bowl, mix low-sodium vegetable broth, tomato paste, dried basil, dried oregano, salt, and pepper to make the kidney-friendly sauce.

5. Pour the sauce over the sautéed vegetables in the skillet. Stir and cook for an additional 2-3 minutes until the sauce thickens slightly.

6. Add chopped spinach and cooked pasta to the skillet. Toss everything together until the pasta and vegetables are evenly coated with the sauce.

7. Remove from heat and serve the Pasta Primavera with Kidney-Friendly Sauce in bowls.

8. Enjoy this colorful and flavorful pasta dish that's kidney-friendly and packed with vegetables!

Nutritional Value (per serving - estimated):

- Calories: 300 kcal
- Protein: 10g
- Fat: 5g
- Carbohydrates: 55g
- Fiber: 8g
- Sodium: 150mg
- Potassium: 360mg

Snacks and Appetizers

Recipe 1: *Hummus with Low-Potassium Veggies*

This Hummus with Low-Potassium Veggies is a nutritious and kidney-friendly snack or appetizer, combining homemade hummus with fresh, low-potassium vegetables.

PREP TIME: 10 MINUTES

COOK TIME: 0 MINUTES

TOTAL TIME: 10 MINUTES

SERVINGS: 4

Ingredients:

- One can of (15 oz) low-sodium chickpeas, drained and rinsed
- 2 tablespoons tahini
- 2 tablespoons lemon juice
- 2 cloves garlic, minced
- 1/4 teaspoon ground cumin
- 2 tablespoons olive oil

- Salt and pepper, to taste
- Low-potassium vegetables for dipping (bell peppers, cucumber slices, etc.)

Instructions:

1. In a food processor, combine drained chickpeas, tahini, lemon juice, minced garlic, ground cumin, olive oil, salt, and pepper.

2. Blend the ingredients until smooth and creamy, scraping down the sides as needed.

3. If the hummus is too thick, add a tablespoon of water at a time and continue blending until desired consistency is achieved.

4. Turn over the hummus to a serving bowl.

5. Wash and prepare low-potassium vegetables like bell peppers or cucumber slices for dipping.

6. Serve the homemade Hummus with Low-Potassium Veggies as a nutritious and kidney-friendly snack or appetizer!

Nutritional Value (per serving - estimated):

- Calories: 180 kcal
- Protein: 7g
- Fat: 10g
- Carbohydrates: 18g
- Fiber: 6g
- Sodium: 120mg
- Potassium: 200mg

Recipe 2: *Roasted Chickpeas*

These Roasted Chickpeas are a crunchy and flavorful snack, perfect for a satisfying munch between meals.

PREP TIME: 5 MINUTES

COOK TIME: 40 MINUTES

TOTAL TIME: 45 MINUTES

SERVINGS: 4

Ingredients:

- 2 cans (15 oz each) chickpeas (garbanzo beans), drained and rinsed
- 2 tablespoons olive oil
- 1 teaspoon paprika
- 1 teaspoon garlic powder
- 1 teaspoon cumin
- Half teaspoon of cayenne pepper (adjust to taste)
- Salt, to taste

Instructions:

1. Preheat the oven to 400°F (200°C). With parchment paper, arrange a baking sheet.

2. Rinse and drain the chickpeas. To remove excess moisture, pat the chickpeas dry with a paper towel

3. In a bowl, toss the dried chickpeas with olive oil, paprika, garlic powder, cumin, cayenne pepper, and salt until evenly coated.

4. Spread the seasoned chickpeas onto the prepared baking sheet in a single layer.

5. Bake in the preheated oven for 30-40 minutes, stirring or shaking the pan occasionally, until the chickpeas are crispy and golden brown.

6. Once done, remove from the oven and let the Roasted Chickpeas cool completely before serving.

7. Enjoy these crispy and flavorful Roasted Chickpeas as a nutritious and satisfying snack!

Nutritional Value (per serving - estimated):

- Calories: 220 kcal
- Protein: 10g
- Fat: 8g
- Carbohydrates: 29g
- Fiber: 8g
- Sodium: 280mg
- Potassium: 320mg

Recipe 3: *Homemade Guacamole with Low-Potassium Chips*

This Homemade Guacamole with Low-Potassium Chips is a flavorful dip paired with low-potassium chips, making it a kidney-friendly snack option.

PREP TIME: 15 MINUTES

COOK TIME: 10 MINUTES (for low-potassium chips, if making from scratch)

TOTAL TIME: 25 MINUTES

SERVINGS: 4

Ingredients:

- 3 ripe avocados, peeled and pitted
- 1 small tomato, diced
- 1/4 cup red onion, finely chopped
- 2 tablespoons fresh cilantro, chopped
- 1-2 tablespoons lime juice
- 1 clove garlic, minced
- Salt and pepper, to taste

- Low-potassium chips (store-bought or homemade)

Instructions:

1. In a mixing bowl, mash the peeled and pitted avocados using a fork or potato masher.

2. Add diced tomato, finely chopped red onion, chopped cilantro, lime juice, minced garlic, salt, and pepper to the mashed avocado. Mix until well combined.

3. Taste and adjust the seasoning or lime juice according to preference.

4. Transfer the Homemade Guacamole to a serving bowl.

5. Serve the guacamole with low-potassium chips for dipping.

6. Enjoy this flavorful Homemade Guacamole with Low-Potassium Chips as a kidney-friendly snack or appetizer!

Nutritional Value (per serving - estimated):

Guacamole (per serving):

- Calories: 170 kcal
- Protein: 3g
- Fat: 15g
- Carbohydrates: 11g
- Fiber: 8g
- Sodium: 10mg
- Potassium: 620mg (estimated)
- Low-Potassium Chips (varies based on type, if homemade)

Recipe 4: Crispy Baked Tofu Bites

These Crispy Baked Tofu Bites are a delightful and protein-rich snack, perfect for satisfying cravings in a healthier way.

PREP TIME: 15 MINUTES

COOK TIME: 25 MINUTES

TOTAL TIME: 40 MINUTES

SERVINGS: 4

Ingredients:

- One block of (14 oz) extra-firm tofu, pressed and drained
- 2 tablespoons cornstarch
- 2 tablespoons nutritional yeast
- 1 teaspoon garlic powder
- 1 teaspoon smoked paprika
- 1/2 teaspoon onion powder
- 1/2 teaspoon salt
- 1/4 teaspoon black pepper
- 2 tablespoons olive oil

Instructions:

1. Preheat the oven to 400°F (200°C). With parchment paper, arrange a baking sheet.

2. Cut the pressed tofu into bite-sized cubes or rectangles.

3. In a bowl, mix together cornstarch, nutritional yeast, garlic powder, smoked paprika, onion powder, salt, and black pepper.

4. Toss the tofu cubes in the dry mixture until evenly coated.

5. Drizzle olive oil over the coated tofu and toss gently to ensure the tofu pieces are coated with oil.

6. Arrange the coated tofu pieces on the prepared baking sheet in a single layer.

7. Bake in the preheated oven for 20-25 minutes, flipping the tofu halfway through, until they are crispy and golden.

8. Once done, remove the Crispy Baked Tofu Bites from the oven and let them cool slightly before serving.

9. Enjoy these flavorful and crunchy tofu bites as a healthy snack or appetizer!

Nutritional Value (per serving - estimated):

- Calories: 180 kcal
- Protein: 12g
- Fat: 10g

- Carbohydrates: 9g
- Fiber: 2g
- Sodium: 300mg
- Potassium: 180mg

Recipe 5: *Vegetable Sticks with Low-Potassium Dip*

This Vegetable Sticks with Low-Potassium Dip is a refreshing and nutritious snack, combining fresh vegetables with a kidney-friendly dip for guilt-free munching.

PREP TIME: 15 MINUTES

COOK TIME: 0 MINUTES

TOTAL TIME: 15 MINUTES

SERVINGS: 4

Ingredients:

- Assorted low-potassium vegetables for sticks (carrots, celery, cucumber, bell peppers, etc.)

Low-potassium dip:

- One cup of low-fat sour cream or Greek yogurt
- 2 tablespoons chopped fresh dill
- 1 tablespoon lemon juice
- 1 clove garlic, minced
- Salt and pepper, to taste

Instructions:

1. Wash, peel (if necessary), and cut the low-potassium vegetables into stick shapes suitable for dipping.

2. In a bowl, mix together low-fat sour cream or Greek yogurt, chopped fresh dill, lemon juice, minced garlic, salt, and pepper to make the low-potassium dip. Adjust seasoning to taste.

3. Transfer the prepared dip to a serving bowl.

4. Arrange the assorted vegetable sticks on a serving platter alongside the low-potassium dip.

5. Serve these Vegetable Sticks with Low-Potassium Dip as a healthy and refreshing snack option!

Nutritional Value (per serving - estimated):

Vegetables (per serving):

- Calories: Varies based on vegetables used
- Protein: Varies
- Fat: Varies
- Carbohydrates: Varies
- Fiber: Varies
- Sodium: Varies
- Potassium: Varies

Dip (per serving):

- Calories: 50 kcal
- Protein: 3g
- Fat: 2g
- Carbohydrates: 5g
- Fiber: 0g
- Sodium: 30mg
- Potassium: 70mg

Dessert Recipes

Recipe 1: *Baked Apple Slices with Cinnamon*

These Baked Apple Slices with Cinnamon are a delightful, naturally sweetened treat, perfect for a healthy dessert or snack.

PREP TIME: 10 MINUTES

COOK TIME: 25 MINUTES

TOTAL TIME: 35 MINUTES

SERVINGS: 2

Ingredients:

- 2 apples, cored and sliced
- 1 tablespoon lemon juice
- One tablespoon of honey or maple syrup this is optional.
- 1 teaspoon ground cinnamon
- 1/2 teaspoon nutmeg (optional)
- 1 tablespoon melted butter or coconut oil (optional)

Instructions:

1. Preheat the oven to 375°F (190°C). With parchment paper, arrange a baking sheet.

2. In a bowl, toss the apple slices with lemon juice to prevent browning.

3. If using, drizzle honey or maple syrup over the apple slices and toss to coat evenly.

4. Sprinkle ground cinnamon (and nutmeg if desired) over the apples and toss to ensure they are coated with the spices.

5. Arrange the coated apple slices in a single layer on the prepared baking sheet.

6. If desired, drizzle melted butter or coconut oil over the apple slices.

7. Bake in the preheated oven for 20-25 minutes until the apples are tender and slightly caramelized.

8. Once done, remove the Baked Apple Slices from the oven and let them cool for a few minutes before serving.

9. Enjoy these warm and aromatic Baked Apple Slices as a delightful dessert or snack!

Nutritional Value (per serving - estimated):

- Calories: 90 kcal
- Protein: 0g
- Fat: 0g
- Carbohydrates: 24g
- Fiber: 4g
- Sodium: 0mg
- Potassium: 190mg

Recipe 2: *Chia Seed Pudding with Low-Potassium Fruits*

This Chia Seed Pudding with Low-Potassium Fruits is a creamy and nutritious dessert or breakfast option, perfect for a kidney-friendly diet.

PREP TIME: 5 MINUTES

CHILL TIME: 4 HOURS OR OVERNIGHT

TOTAL TIME: 4 HOURS 5 MINUTES (including chill time)

SERVINGS: 2

Ingredients:

- 1/4 cup chia seeds
- One cup of unsweetened almond milk or any low-potassium milk alternative
- One tablespoon of honey or maple syrup this is optional.
- 1/2 teaspoon vanilla extract
- Low-potassium fruits for topping (such as berries, mango, or peaches)

Instructions:

1. In a bowl or jar, combine chia seeds, unsweetened almond milk (or your choice of low-potassium milk), honey or maple syrup (if using), and vanilla extract. Mix well.

2. Stir the mixture vigorously to prevent clumping of chia seeds. Ensure all the chia seeds are fully submerged in the liquid.

3. Cover the bowl or jar and refrigerate for at least 4 hours or overnight, allowing the chia seeds to absorb the liquid and form a pudding-like consistency.

4. Once the chia seed pudding has set, divide it into serving bowls or glasses.

5. Top the Chia Seed Pudding with Low-Potassium Fruits of your choice, such as berries, mango slices, or diced peaches.

6. Serve this nutritious and flavorful Chia Seed Pudding with Low-Potassium Fruits as a delicious dessert or breakfast option!

Nutritional Value (per serving - estimated):

Chia Seed Pudding (per serving):

- Calories: 120 kcal
- Protein: 4g
- Fat: 7g
- Carbohydrates: 12g
- Fiber: 9g
- Sodium: 80mg
- Potassium: 100mg (estimated)

Recipe 3: Vegan Banana Bread

This Vegan Banana Bread is moist, flavorful, and a perfect way to utilize ripe bananas, making it a delightful treat for any occasion.

PREP TIME: 15 MINUTES

COOK TIME: 50-60 MINUTES

TOTAL TIME: 1 HOUR 5 MINUTES - 1 HOUR 15 MINUTES

SERVINGS: 10

Ingredients:

- 3 ripe bananas, mashed
- 1/3 cup coconut oil, melted
- Half cup of maple syrup or agave nectar
- 1/4 cup plant-based milk (such as almond or oat milk)
- 1 teaspoon vanilla extract
- 1 3/4 cups of all-purpose flour or whole wheat flour
- 1 teaspoon baking soda
- 1/2 teaspoon ground cinnamon
- 1/4 teaspoon salt
- (Optional) add-ins e.g. chopped nuts, chocolate chips, or dried fruits

Instructions:

1. Preheat the oven to 350°F (175°C). Grease or line a loaf pan with parchment paper.

2. In a mixing bowl, combine mashed bananas, melted coconut oil, maple syrup or agave nectar, plant-based milk, and vanilla extract. Mix until well combined.

3. Whisk together the flour, baking soda, ground cinnamon, and salt in a separate bowl.

4. Mix the dry ingredients to the wet ingredients and stir until just combined. Be careful not to overmix.

5. If using, fold in chopped nuts, chocolate chips, or dried fruits into the batter.

6. In the prepared loaf pan, pour in the batter and spread evenly.

7. Until a toothpick inserted into the center comes out clean, keep baking in the preheated oven for fifty to sixty minutes.

8. Once done, remove the Vegan Banana Bread from the oven and allow it to cool in the pan for 10-15 minutes before transferring to a wire rack to cool completely.

9. Slice and enjoy this delicious, moist Vegan Banana Bread as a delightful snack or dessert!

Nutritional Value (per serving - estimated):

- Calories: 220 kcal
- Protein: 2g
- Fat: 9g
- Carbohydrates: 34g
- Fiber: 2g
- Sodium: 150mg
- Potassium: 190mg

Recipe 4: *Coconut Milk Ice Cream with Berries*

This Coconut Milk Ice Cream with Berries is a dairy-free and refreshing dessert, perfect for a sweet treat without compromising on flavor.

PREP TIME: 5 MINUTES

CHURN TIME: 20-25 MINUTES

TOTAL TIME: 25-30 MINUTES

SERVINGS: 4

Ingredients:

- Two cans of (14 oz each) coconut milk (full-fat)
- Half cup of maple syrup or agave nectar
- 1 teaspoon vanilla extract
- One cup of mixed berries e.g. strawberries, blueberries, raspberries
- Fresh mint leaves (for garnish, optional)

Instructions:

1. Place the cans of coconut milk in the refrigerator overnight to chill.

2. In a bowl, whisk together the chilled coconut milk (scooping out the solidified coconut cream on top), maple syrup or agave nectar, and vanilla extract until well combined.

3. Ensure it reaches a soft-serve consistency. But firstly, pour the mixture into an ice cream maker and churn according to the manufacturer's instructions.

4. In the last few minutes of churning, add the mixed berries into the ice cream and allow them to mix evenly.

5. Transfer the Coconut Milk Ice Cream with Berries into a freezer-safe container and freeze for an additional 2-3 hours or until it reaches the desired firmness.

6. When ready to serve, scoop the coconut milk ice cream into bowls or cones.

7. Garnish with additional fresh berries and mint leaves if desired.

8. Enjoy this creamy and dairy-free Coconut Milk Ice Cream with Berries as a delightful dessert!

Nutritional Value (per serving - estimated):

- Calories: 320 kcal
- Protein: 2g
- Fat: 24g
- Carbohydrates: 30g
- Fiber: 2g
- Sodium: 20mg

- Potassium: 280mg

Recipe 5: *Almond Flour Cookies*

These Almond Flour Cookies are a delightful gluten-free and low-carb treat, perfect for satisfying a sweet craving without compromising on flavor.

PREP TIME: 15 MINUTES

COOK TIME: 12-15 MINUTES

TOTAL TIME: 27-30 MINUTES

SERVINGS: 12-15 cookies

Ingredients:

- 2 cups almond flour
- 1/4 cup coconut oil, melted
- 1/4 cup maple syrup or honey
- 1 teaspoon vanilla extract
- 1/4 teaspoon baking soda
- Pinch of salt

- Optional add-ins: chopped dark chocolate, dried fruits, nuts

Instructions:

1. Preheat the oven to 350°F (175°C). With parchment paper, arrange a baking sheet.

2. In a mixing bowl, combine almond flour, melted coconut oil, maple syrup or honey, vanilla extract, baking soda, and a pinch of salt. Mix until a dough forms.

3. If desired, add chopped dark chocolate, dried fruits, nuts, or any other add-ins into the dough and mix until evenly distributed.

4. Using a spoon or cookie scoop, portion out the cookie dough and place them onto the prepared baking sheet. Slightly flatten each cookie with your fingers or the back of a spoon.

5. Until the edges are golden brown, keep baking in the preheated oven for twelve to fifteen minutes.

6. Once done, remove the Almond Flour Cookies from the oven and let them cool on the baking sheet for a few minutes before transferring to a wire rack to cool completely.

7. Enjoy these delicious, gluten-free Almond Flour Cookies as a guilt-free snack or dessert!

Nutritional Value (per serving - estimated for 1 cookie):

- Calories: 120 kcal
- Protein: 3g
- Fat: 9g
- Carbohydrates: 8g
- Fiber: 1g
- Sodium: 40mg
- Potassium: 40mg

Beverages

Recipe 1: *Herbal Tea Infusions (like Chamomile or Peppermint)*

Herbal Tea Infusions like Chamomile or Peppermint are soothing, aromatic, and perfect for relaxation and overall wellness.

PREP TIME: 5 MINUTES

BREW TIME: 5-7 MINUTES

TOTAL TIME: 10-12 MINUTES

SERVINGS: 1 cup per infusion

Ingredients:

- 1 herbal tea bag (Chamomile, Peppermint, or any preferred herbal tea)
- Hot water
- Optional add-ins: honey, lemon slices, fresh mint leaves

Instructions:

1. Pour water in a kettle or saucepan and boil.

2. Place the herbal tea bag (Chamomile, Peppermint, or your preferred herbal tea) in a cup or mug.

3. Pour the hot water over the tea bag, ensuring it's fully submerged.

4. Cover the cup with a saucer or small plate and let the tea steep for 5-7 minutes to allow the flavors to infuse.

5. Once the desired steeping time is reached, remove the tea bag from the cup.

6. If desired, add a drizzle of honey, a few lemon slices, or fresh mint leaves for added flavor.

7. Stir gently and let it cool slightly before sipping and enjoying the soothing and aromatic Herbal Tea Infusion.

8. Relax and unwind with this comforting cup of herbal tea!

Note: Adjust the steeping time based on the herbal tea's recommended brewing time for optimal flavor.

Nutritional Value: (depends on the herbal tea used, typically zero calories and no significant macronutrients)

Recipe 2: *Caffeine-Free Fruit Infused Water*

This Caffeine-Free Fruit Infused Water is a refreshing and hydrating beverage infused with natural flavors, making it an ideal option for staying hydrated throughout the day.

PREP TIME: 5 MINUTES

INFUSION TIME: 2-4 HOURS

TOTAL TIME: 2-4 HOURS 5 MINUTES - 4 HOURS 5 MINUTES

SERVINGS: 4

Ingredients:

- 1-2 fruits of your choice (examples: lemon, lime, orange, berries, cucumber)
- Fresh herbs this is optional, such as mint, basil.
- 8-10 cups water

- Ice cubes (optional)

Instructions:

1. Wash the fruits thoroughly. If using citrus fruits like lemon, lime, or orange, slice them thinly. For berries, crush or slightly muddle them to release flavors. For cucumber, slice thinly.

2. In a large pitcher or container, add the prepared fruits and fresh herbs (if using).

3. Pour cold water over the fruits and herbs in the pitcher.

4. Cover the pitcher and place it in the refrigerator for 2-4 hours to allow the flavors to infuse into the water.

5. Once the fruit-infused water has infused to your liking, remove it from the refrigerator.

6. Serve the Caffeine-Free Fruit Infused Water over ice if desired, and enjoy this refreshing and flavorful beverage!

Note: You can refill the pitcher with water a couple of times before replacing the fruits for additional servings.

Nutritional Value: (depends on the fruits and herbs used, typically minimal calories and no significant macronutrients)

Recipe 3: *Almond Milk or Rice Milk*

Homemade Almond Milk or Rice Milk is a dairy-free alternative that's creamy, versatile, and perfect for various culinary uses or as a standalone beverage.

PREP TIME: 8-12 HOURS (SOAKING) + 5 MINUTES

TOTAL TIME: 8-12 HOURS 5 MINUTES - 12 HOURS 5 MINUTES

SERVINGS: Approx. 4 cups

Ingredients:

For Almond Milk:

- 1 cup raw almonds
- 4 cups water

- Sweetener of choice (optional): dates, honey, or maple syrup
- Vanilla extract (optional)

For Rice Milk:

- One cup of uncooked rice (white or brown)
- 4 cups water
- Sweetener of choice (optional): dates, honey, or maple syrup
- Vanilla extract (optional)

Instructions:

For Almond Milk:

1. Soak raw almonds in water overnight or for at least 8-12 hours.

2. Drain and rinse the almonds thoroughly after soaking.

3. In a blender, combine soaked almonds and 4 cups of fresh water.

4. Blend on high speed for 1-2 minutes until the mixture becomes smooth and creamy.

5. Strain the almond mixture through a nut milk bag, cheesecloth, or fine-mesh sieve into a bowl or pitcher, squeezing out as much liquid as possible.

6. If desired, add sweetener of choice (dates, honey, or maple syrup) and a splash of vanilla extract to the strained almond milk. Stir well.

7. Store the Almond Milk in a sealed container in the refrigerator for up to 3-4 days. Shake well before each use.

For Rice Milk:

1. Rinse the uncooked rice thoroughly.

2. In a blender, combine rinsed rice and 4 cups of fresh water.

3. Blend on high speed for 2-3 minutes until the mixture becomes smooth.

4. Strain the rice mixture through a nut milk bag, cheesecloth, or fine-mesh sieve into a bowl or pitcher, removing any excess sediment.

5. If desired, add sweetener of choice (dates, honey, or maple syrup) and a splash of vanilla extract to the strained rice milk. Stir well.

6. Store the Rice Milk in a sealed container in the refrigerator for up to 3-4 days. Shake well before each use.

Nutritional Value: (per serving - estimated for 1 cup) varies based on added sweeteners or flavorings

Recipe 4: *Low-Potassium Smoothie (Cucumber, Spinach, and Berries)*

This Low-Potassium Smoothie is a nutritious blend of cucumber, spinach, and berries, providing a refreshing and kidney-friendly option packed with vitamins and antioxidants.

PREP TIME: 5 MINUTES

BLEND TIME: 2-3 MINUTES

TOTAL TIME: 7-8 MINUTES

SERVINGS: 2

Ingredients:

- 1 cup cucumber, peeled and chopped
- 1 cup fresh spinach leaves
- Half cup of mixed berries e.g. strawberries, blueberries, raspberries.
- 1/2 cup low-potassium liquid (such as almond milk or apple juice)
- 1/2 cup ice cubes (optional)
- Sweetener of choice (optional): honey or maple syrup

Instructions:

1. In a blender, combine the chopped cucumber, fresh spinach leaves, mixed berries, and low-potassium liquid (almond milk or apple juice).

2. If desired, add ice cubes for a chilled smoothie.

3. Blend on high speed for 2-3 minutes or until the mixture becomes smooth and well combined.

4. Taste the smoothie and add a sweetener like honey or maple syrup if desired. To incorporate well, blend again for a Few seconds.

5. Once blended to your desired consistency, pour the Low-Potassium Smoothie into glasses.

6. Serve immediately and enjoy this nutritious and kidney-friendly smoothie!

Nutritional Value (per serving - estimated):

- Calories: 50 kcal
- Protein: 1g
- Fat: 0.5g
- Carbohydrates: 12g
- Fiber: 3g
- Sodium: 20mg
- Potassium: 150mg (estimated)

Recipe 5: *Freshly Squeezed Apple Juice*

This Freshly Squeezed Apple Juice is a simple and delicious beverage that's naturally sweet and refreshing, perfect for a potassium-friendly drink.

PREP TIME: 10 MINUTES

TOTAL TIME: 10 MINUTES

SERVINGS: 2

Ingredients:

- 4-5 apples (any variety), washed and cored

Instructions:

1. Wash the apples thoroughly, then core and slice them into smaller pieces.

2. Using a juicer or a blender, extract the juice from the apples. If using a blender, blend the apple pieces until smooth and strain the juice using a fine-mesh sieve or cheesecloth to remove pulp.

3. Collect the freshly squeezed apple juice in a pitcher or bowl.

4. Stir the juice to ensure it's well combined and serve immediately.

5. Optionally, you can chill the apple juice in the refrigerator for a refreshing cold drink.

6. Enjoy this Freshly Squeezed Apple Juice as a delightful and potassium-friendly beverage!

Nutritional Value (per serving - estimated):

- Calories: 120 kcal
- Protein: 0g
- Fat: 0g
- Carbohydrates: 30g
- Fiber: 4g
- Sodium: 0mg
- Potassium: 200mg (estimated)

Congratulations if you have followed these mouthwatering renal friendly recipes to this point, these meals are specially crafted to provide your kidneys with the necessary nutrients needed to boost its function. As you incorporate these meals into your daily lives, never forget to keep an eye on your portion size. In the next phase of this book (bonus section), we will delve into a specially crafted 28-day meal plan to help your healthy eating journey. You will also be provided with a meal tracker to help you monitor and use the recipes in this book appropriately

Bonus 1

28- day meal plan

I welcome you to a 28-day meal plan, meticulously crafted to provide your kidneys with the desired nutrition for optimal performance. Endeavor you follow this plan accordingly and always keep an eye on portion sizes

Week 1:

Day 1:

- Breakfast: Quinoa Breakfast Bowl
- Lunch: Chickpea Salad Wraps
- Dinner: Baked Herb-Crusted Tofu with Steamed Vegetables

Day 2:

- Breakfast: Vegetable Omelette with Spinach and Peppers
- Lunch: Zucchini Noodles with Pesto Sauce
- Dinner: Eggplant and Tomato Casserole

Day 3:

- Breakfast: Almond Flour Pancakes with Berries
- Lunch: Black Bean and Vegetable Burrito Bowl
- Dinner: Cauliflower Rice Stir-Fry with Tofu or Tempeh

Day 4:

- Breakfast: Chia Seed Pudding with Low-Potassium Fruits
- Lunch: Lentil and Vegetable Soup
- Dinner: Vegan Lentil Shepherd's Pie

Day 5:

- Breakfast: Avocado Toast with Low-Potassium Toppings
- Lunch: Pasta Primavera with Kidney-Friendly Sauce
- Dinner: Mushroom and Spinach Quinoa Salad

Day 6:

- Breakfast: Freshly Squeezed Apple Juice
- Lunch: Hummus with Low-Potassium Veggies
- Dinner: Baked Apple Slices with Cinnamon

Day 7:

- Breakfast: Low-Potassium Smoothie (Cucumber, Spinach, and Berries)
- Lunch: Vegetable Sticks with Low-Potassium Dip
- Dinner: Crispy Baked Tofu Bites

Week 2:

Day 8:

- Breakfast: Vegan Banana Bread
- Lunch: Baked Black Bean and Vegetable Burritos
- Dinner: Pasta Primavera with Kidney-Friendly Sauce

Day 9:

- Breakfast: Quinoa Breakfast Bowl
- Lunch: Lentil and Vegetable Soup
- Dinner: Eggplant and Tomato Casserole

Day 10:

- Breakfast: Almond Flour Cookies
- Lunch: Chickpea Salad Wraps
- Dinner: Zucchini Noodles with Pesto Sauce

Day 11:

- Breakfast: Chia Seed Pudding with Low-Potassium Fruits
- Lunch: Mushroom and Spinach Quinoa Salad
- Dinner: Vegan Lentil Shepherd's Pie

Day 12:

- Breakfast: Avocado Toast with Low-Potassium Toppings
- Lunch: Hummus with Low-Potassium Veggies
- Dinner: Cauliflower Rice Stir-Fry with Tofu or Tempeh

Day 13:

- Breakfast: Freshly Squeezed Apple Juice
- Lunch: Vegetable Sticks with Low-Potassium Dip
- Dinner: Baked Apple Slices with Cinnamon

Day 14:

- Breakfast: Low-Potassium Smoothie (Cucumber, Spinach, and Berries)
- Lunch: Crispy Baked Tofu Bites
- Dinner: Herbal Tea Infusions (like Chamomile or Peppermint)

Week 3:

Day 15:

- Breakfast: Almond Flour Pancakes with Berries
- Lunch: Black Bean and Vegetable Burrito Bowl
- Dinner: Baked Herb-Crusted Tofu with Steamed Vegetables

Day 16:

- Breakfast: Vegetable Omelette with Spinach and Peppers

- Lunch: Lentil and Vegetable Soup
- Dinner: Eggplant and Tomato Casserole

Day 17:

- Breakfast: Vegan Banana Bread
- Lunch: Chickpea Salad Wraps
- Dinner: Zucchini Noodles with Pesto Sauce

Day 18:

- Breakfast: Chia Seed Pudding with Low-Potassium Fruits
- Lunch: Mushroom and Spinach Quinoa Salad
- Dinner: Vegan Lentil Shepherd's Pie

Day 19:

- Breakfast: Avocado Toast with Low-Potassium Toppings
- Lunch: Hummus with Low-Potassium Veggies

- Dinner: Cauliflower Rice Stir-Fry with Tofu or Tempeh

Day 20:

- Breakfast: Freshly Squeezed Apple Juice
- Lunch: Vegetable Sticks with Low-Potassium Dip
- Dinner: Baked Apple Slices with Cinnamon

Day 21:

- Breakfast: Low-Potassium Smoothie (Cucumber, Spinach, and Berries)
- Lunch: Crispy Baked Tofu Bites
- Dinner: Herbal Tea Infusions (like Chamomile or Peppermint)

Week 4:

Day 22:

- Breakfast: Quinoa Breakfast Bowl
- Lunch: Baked Black Bean and Vegetable Burritos
- Dinner: Pasta Primavera with Kidney-Friendly Sauce

Day 23:

- Breakfast: Vegan Banana Bread
- Lunch: Lentil and Vegetable Soup
- Dinner: Eggplant and Tomato Casserole

Day 24:

- Breakfast: Almond Flour Cookies
- Lunch: Chickpea Salad Wraps
- Dinner: Zucchini Noodles with Pesto Sauce

Day 25:

- Breakfast: Chia Seed Pudding with Low-Potassium Fruits
- Lunch: Mushroom and Spinach Quinoa Salad
- Dinner: Vegan Lentil Shepherd's Pie

Day 26:

- Breakfast: Avocado Toast with Low-Potassium Toppings
- Lunch: Hummus with Low-Potassium Veggies
- Dinner: Cauliflower Rice Stir-Fry with Tofu or Tempeh

Day 27:

- Breakfast: Freshly Squeezed Apple Juice
- Lunch: Vegetable Sticks with Low-Potassium Dip
- Dinner: Baked Apple Slices with Cinnamon

Day 28:

- Breakfast: Low-Potassium Smoothie (Cucumber, Spinach, and Berries)
- Lunch: Crispy Baked Tofu Bites
- Dinner: Herbal Tea Infusions (like Chamomile or Peppermint)

Bonus 2

Meal Journal

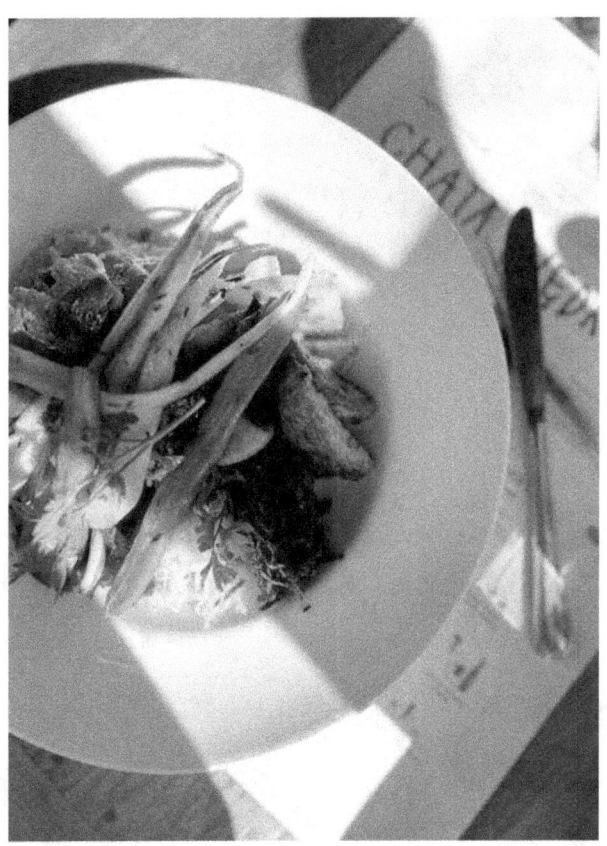

FOOD JOURNAL

Breakfast	Servings	Calories
	Subtotal	

Snack		
	Subtotal	

Lunch		
	Subtotal	

Snack		
	Subtotal	

Dinner		
	Subtotal	

Snack		
	Subtotal	

Total Calories From Food [   ]

FITNESS ACTIVITY JOURNAL

	Duration	Calories

Total Calories From Fitness [   ]

NOTES

_____

_____

_____

_____

_____

_____

FOOD JOURNAL

Breakfast	Servings	Calories
	Subtotal	

Snack		
	Subtotal	

Lunch		
	Subtotal	

Snack		
	Subtotal	

Dinner		
	Subtotal	

Snack		
	Subtotal	
Total Calories From Food		

FITNESS ACTIVITY JOURNAL

	Duration	Calories
Total Calories From Fitness		

NOTES

FOOD JOURNAL

Breakfast	Servings	Calories
		Subtotal

Snack		
		Subtotal

Lunch		
		Subtotal

Snack		
		Subtotal

Dinner		
		Subtotal

Snack		
		Subtotal

Total Calories From Food

FITNESS ACTIVITY JOURNAL

	Duration	Calories

Total Calories From Fitness

NOTES

FOOD JOURNAL

Breakfast	Servings	Calories
	Subtotal	

Snack		
	Subtotal	

Lunch		
	Subtotal	

Snack		
	Subtotal	

Dinner		
	Subtotal	

Snack		
	Subtotal	
	Total Calories From Food	

FITNESS ACTIVITY JOURNAL

	Duration	Calories
	Total Calories From Fitness	

NOTES

FOOD JOURNAL

Breakfast	Servings	Calories
	Subtotal	

Snack		
	Subtotal	

Lunch		
	Subtotal	

Snack		
	Subtotal	

Dinner		
	Subtotal	

Snack		
	Subtotal	

Total Calories From Food	

FITNESS ACTIVITY JOURNAL

	Duration	Calories

Total Calories From Fitness	

NOTES

FOOD JOURNAL

Breakfast	Servings	Calories
	Subtotal	

Snack		
	Subtotal	

Lunch		
	Subtotal	

Snack		
	Subtotal	

Dinner		
	Subtotal	

Snack		
	Subtotal	

Total Calories From Food [　　　　　　]

FITNESS ACTIVITY JOURNAL

	Duration	Calories

Total Calories From Fitness [　　　　　　]

NOTES

_____

_____

_____

_____

_____

FOOD JOURNAL

Breakfast	Servings	Calories
		Subtotal

Snack		
		Subtotal

Lunch		
		Subtotal

Snack		
		Subtotal

Dinner		
		Subtotal

Snack		
		Subtotal
Total Calories From Food		

FITNESS ACTIVITY JOURNAL

	Duration	Calories
Total Calories From Fitness		

NOTES

FOOD JOURNAL

Breakfast	Servings	Calories
		Subtotal

Snack		
		Subtotal

Lunch		
		Subtotal

Snack		
		Subtotal

Dinner		
		Subtotal

Snack		
		Subtotal

Total Calories From Food

FITNESS ACTIVITY JOURNAL

	Duration	Calories

Total Calories From Fitness

NOTES

FOOD JOURNAL

Breakfast	Servings	Calories
	Subtotal	

Snack		
	Subtotal	

Lunch		
	Subtotal	

Snack		
	Subtotal	

Dinner		
	Subtotal	

Snack		
	Subtotal	
Total Calories From Food		

FITNESS ACTIVITY JOURNAL

	Duration	Calories
Total Calories From Fitness		

NOTES

FOOD JOURNAL

Breakfast	Servings	Calories
	Subtotal	
Snack		
	Subtotal	
Lunch		
	Subtotal	
Snack		
	Subtotal	
Dinner		
	Subtotal	
Snack		
	Subtotal	
	Total Calories From Food	

FITNESS ACTIVITY JOURNAL

	Duration	Calories
	Total Calories From Fitness	

NOTES

FOOD JOURNAL

Breakfast	Servings	Calories
	Subtotal	

Snack		
	Subtotal	

Lunch		
	Subtotal	

Snack		
	Subtotal	

Dinner		
	Subtotal	

Snack		
	Subtotal	

Total Calories From Food

FITNESS ACTIVITY JOURNAL

	Duration	Calories

Total Calories From Fitness

NOTES

FOOD JOURNAL

Breakfast	Servings	Calories
	Subtotal	

Snack		
	Subtotal	

Lunch		
	Subtotal	

Snack		
	Subtotal	

Dinner		
	Subtotal	

Snack		
	Subtotal	

Total Calories From Food

FITNESS ACTIVITY JOURNAL

	Duration	Calories

Total Calories From Fitness

NOTES

FOOD JOURNAL

Breakfast	Servings	Calories
	Subtotal	

Snack		
	Subtotal	

Lunch		
	Subtotal	

Snack		
	Subtotal	

Dinner		
	Subtotal	

Snack		
	Subtotal	
	Total Calories From Food	

FITNESS ACTIVITY JOURNAL

	Duration	Calories
	Total Calories From Fitness	

NOTES

_____

_____

_____

_____

_____

_____

FOOD JOURNAL

Breakfast	Servings	Calories
	Subtotal	

Snack		
	Subtotal	

Lunch		
	Subtotal	

Snack		
	Subtotal	

Dinner		
	Subtotal	

Snack		
	Subtotal	
Total Calories From Food		

FITNESS ACTIVITY JOURNAL

	Duration	Calories
Total Calories From Fitness		

NOTES

FOOD JOURNAL

Breakfast	Servings	Calories
	Subtotal	

Snack		
	Subtotal	

Lunch		
	Subtotal	

Snack		
	Subtotal	

Dinner		
	Subtotal	

Snack		
	Subtotal	

Total Calories From Food

FITNESS ACTIVITY JOURNAL

	Duration	Calories

Total Calories From Fitness

NOTES

FOOD JOURNAL

Breakfast	Servings	Calories
	Subtotal	

Snack		
	Subtotal	

Lunch		
	Subtotal	

Snack		
	Subtotal	

Dinner		
	Subtotal	

Snack		
	Subtotal	

Total Calories From Food [ ]

FITNESS ACTIVITY JOURNAL

	Duration	Calories

Total Calories From Fitness [ ]

NOTES

FOOD JOURNAL

Breakfast	Servings	Calories
	Subtotal	

Snack		
	Subtotal	

Lunch		
	Subtotal	

Snack		
	Subtotal	

Dinner		
	Subtotal	

Snack		
	Subtotal	

Total Calories From Food [   ]

FITNESS ACTIVITY JOURNAL

	Duration	Calories

Total Calories From Fitness [   ]

NOTES

FOOD JOURNAL

Breakfast	Servings	Calories
	Subtotal	

Snack		
	Subtotal	

Lunch		
	Subtotal	

Snack		
	Subtotal	

Dinner		
	Subtotal	

Snack		
	Subtotal	

Total Calories From Food

FITNESS ACTIVITY JOURNAL

	Duration	Calories

Total Calories From Fitness

NOTES

FOOD JOURNAL

Breakfast	Servings	Calories
	Subtotal	

Snack		
	Subtotal	

Lunch		
	Subtotal	

Snack		
	Subtotal	

Dinner		
	Subtotal	

Snack		
	Subtotal	
	Total Calories From Food	

FITNESS ACTIVITY JOURNAL

	Duration	Calories
	Total Calories From Fitness	

NOTES

Conclusion

Dear Readers, as we draw to the end of this book, here is a recap;

Throughout our conversation and exploration of the *"Chronic Kidney Disease Stage 3 Cookbook for Women,"* the central theme has been empowerment through nutrition. Managing Chronic Kidney Disease (CKD) Stage 3 may initially seem daunting, but this cookbook is a beacon of hope, guidance, and reassurance.

Living with CKD Stage 3 can be challenging, but this cookbook is a testament to the notion that delicious, nourishing meals can be a cornerstone of managing this condition. It offers a wealth of recipes specially crafted to cater to the dietary needs of women navigating this journey. Remember, every meal you prepare using these recipes is a step towards supporting your kidney health and overall well-being.

It's natural to have doubts or fears when facing a condition like CKD Stage 3. However, this cookbook serves not only as a recipe collection but also as a guide addressing concerns. From exploring the biochemistry behind the condition to outlining risk factors and symptoms, it offers comprehensive insights to help demystify and empower individuals facing CKD Stage 3.

Navigating dietary restrictions can be overwhelming, but this cookbook eliminates the fear of bland or tasteless meals. It showcases a diverse array of flavorful recipes, ensuring that your journey towards wellness is both delicious and satisfying. With meal plans, shopping lists, and practical tips, this book makes the process seamless.

Food is more than mere sustenance; it's a powerful tool for healing and vitality. This cookbook embodies the belief that adopting a kidney-friendly diet doesn't mean sacrificing taste or variety. It's a celebration of flavors, offering a roadmap to nourishment and wellness.

As you embark on this culinary journey, remember that every small step towards healthier eating habits counts. Embrace this opportunity to take charge of your health, knowing that with each meal prepared from this cookbook, you're nurturing your body and supporting your kidneys.

Together, let's foster a mindset of wellness, resilience, and empowerment. You're not alone in this journey. With the right knowledge, support, and flavorful recipes in hand, you have the tools to navigate CKD Stage 3 with confidence and optimism.

Remember, your health is a priority. Embrace the nourishing power of food and savor the journey towards a healthier, happier you.

Appreciation

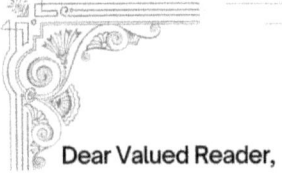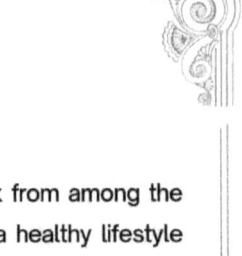

Dear Valued Reader,

Thank you for selecting our cookbook from among the many available. Your decision to live a healthy lifestyle with the help of our book means everything to us. We welcome you to share your thoughts on the website by leaving a polite review. Your feedback supports our journey, and we are grateful. Let your words be the heartbeat of our collective dedication to happiness. We also humbly request that you visit and follow our author page; by doing so, you will be exposed to a plethora of other publications by this author.

With appreciation,

DR. LUNA O. RICHARDS

CHECK OUT OTHER BOOKS FROM THE AUTHOR

You can kindly check out some other books on kidney disease by this author. Click the respective book links below to get a copy of these books, or scan the QR Codes to gain access.

Chronic Kidney Disease Stage 3 Cookbook for Men

Kidney Disease Diet Stage 3 Cookbook

Chronic Kidney Disease Stage 3 Cookbook for Beginners

 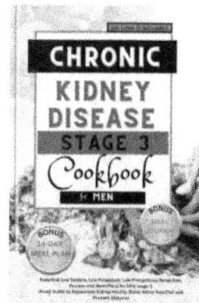

Scan the Code to get the Chronic Kidney
Disease Stage 3 Cookbook for Men

 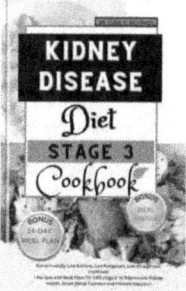

Scan the Code to get the Kidney Disease Stage 3
Cookbook

 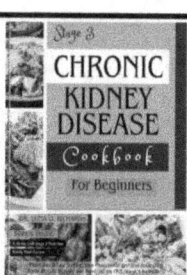

Scan the Code to get the Chronic Kidney Disease
Stage 3 Cookbook for Beginners

 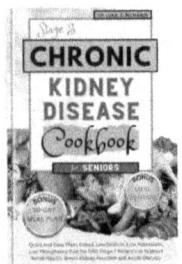

Scan the Code to get the Chronic Kidney Disease
Stage 3 Cookbook for Seniors

ACKNOWLEDGEMENT

Picture Links

https://www.freepik.com/free-photo/view-bowl-with-shells-arrangement_12349144.htm

https://www.freepik.com/free-photo/composition-noodles-table_11741223.htm

https://www.freepik.com/free-photo/beautiful-young-woman-cutting-fresh-vegetables-kitchen_1624303.htm